Action Research in Health

Ernest Stringer, Ph.D.

William Genat, Ph.D.

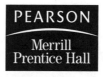

PEARSON

Merrill
Prentice Hall

Upper Saddle River, New Jersey
Columbus, Ohio

Library of Congress Cataloging-in-Publication Data

Stringer, Ernest T.
  Action research in health/Ernie Stringer, William J. Genat.
    p. cm.
  Includes bibliographical references and index.
  ISBN 0-13-098578-3
    1. Action research. 2. Medical care—Research—Methodology. 3. Action research in
public health. I. Genat, William J. II. Title.

RA440.85.S776 2004
362.1'072—dc21   2003056128

Vice President and Executive Publisher: Jeffery W. Johnston
Publisher: Kevin M. Davis
Editorial Assistant: Autumn Crisp
Production Editor: Mary Harlan
Production Coordinator: Lea Baranowski, Carlisle Publishers Services
Design Coordinator: Diane C. Lorenzo
Text Design and Illustrations: Carlisle Publishers Services
Cover Design: Rod Harris
Cover Image: Getty One
Production Manager: Laura Messerly
Director of Marketing: Ann Castel Davis
Marketing Manager: Amy June
Marketing Coordinator: Tyra Poole

This book was set in Century Light by Carlisle Communications, Ltd. It was printed and bound by
R. R. Donnelley & Sons Company. The cover was printed by Phoenix Color Corp.

Pearson Education Ltd.   Pearson Education Australia Pty. Limited
Pearson Education Singapore Pte. Ltd.   Pearson Education North Asia Ltd.
Pearson Education Canada, Ltd.   Pearson Educación de Mexico, S.A. de C.V.
Pearson Education–Japan   Pearson Education Malaysia Pte. Ltd.

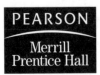

10 9 8 7 6 5 4 3 2 1
ISBN: 0-13-098578-3

Preface

Introduction

Action research is a rigorous and systematic approach to investigation that integrates the expertise of professionals and the local wisdom of the people they serve. This book provides step-by-step procedures for enacting research processes that, to some extent, run across the grain of the carefully prescribed, objective routines of experimental research that historically have been the hallmark of medical research. The purpose of this book is to show how health professionals can make more effective use of their expertise by ensuring that it "makes sense" to their clients, while providing the basis for health care that is easily integrated into the home, work, and/or community life of the individuals concerned.

This book represents the outcome of twenty years of experience working with each other and like-minded associates. Our task has been to find ways to ensure that the collective wisdom and insight of local people informs the programs and services meant to enhance their health and well-being. Over the years, both of us have witnessed caring and committed professionals who, in managing the multiple demands on their time, often paid little heed to client perspectives. One example of the often futile interventions of the all-knowing health professional is provided by the story of one of our colleagues. A wonderfully passionate doctor, he went to Yemen as a very young man, and became absorbed in the task of working to enhance the health status of the local people. With an eye to the preventive side of public health, in particular, nutrition and income support, Peter imported a herd of goats for the benefit of the locals. Years later, he now recounts the story of how the whole herd was lost to altitude sickness.

Such tales emphasize the way unaccounted subtleties of local circumstances, culture, or geography may undermine the good intentions of those working in the health arena. The effects of globalization and the multicultural nature of many urban and suburban contexts challenge health professionals to find ways of ensuring that their carefully prescribed programs of care can be implemented effectively in the lives of their clients. One of the central premises of this book, therefore, is that local people themselves must participate in the investigations and plans that provide the basis for health care.

Our collective experience enacting action research covers a wide range of contexts and includes projects undertaken in university, institutional, and community settings. They include urban, rural, and remote locations in both developed and lesser developed nations and frequently incorporate multidisciplinary teams. A key feature of all these action research projects has been not only the learning gained by the participants themselves but also our learning about methods of practice. In these pages we seek to share the gift bestowed upon us by others we have worked with.

Our experience suggests that the enactment of action research has placed us in uniquely special and privileged positions. In bringing together diverse groups of participants, we often find ourselves creating a special kind of social space where people feel safe and comfortable enough to share stories about their lives. The experience is sometimes quite emotional, sometimes even exciting and liberating for the storyteller, and often extremely informative for both speaker and listener. It is this rich kind of engagement that we both have been privileged to experience within our work.

The Nature of the Book

Action research differs from the forms of experimental and quasi-experimental research that have historically dominated the health arena. While action research will continue to contribute to the general body of objective knowledge that informs the practice of health professionals, its major purpose is to seek practical solutions to problems in particular contexts. In doing so, it engages participants in subjective routines of inquiry and investigation that provide forms of understanding specifically relevant to the situation of clients and enables the most effective use of knowledge available from the biomedical sciences. Action research is based on the premise that health care is most effective when it is consciously engaged in ways meaningful to clients and easily integrated into day-to-day life. Action research, therefore, is presented as a way in which the expertise and knowledge of the health professional complements the "common-sense," cultural knowledge people have of their everyday lives.

Chapters 1 and 2 describe action research as a mode of investigation, and seek to clarify how action research differs from other forms of research.

Chapters 3 through 6 provide a detailed description of action research, taking readers through one research cycle from framing and focusing the investigation to reporting and communicating the outcomes of the process.

Chapter 7 provides examples of common professional practice routines, suggesting how systematic processes of investigation can be incorporated into a health professional's daily activities.

Chapter 8 presents a number of examples of the way action research has been successfully applied to a range of problems in a number of different contexts.

Chapter 9 lists of some of the Websites that can link health professionals to the vast resources now available on the World Wide Web.

Acknowledgments

Over the years, colleagues from widely diverse disciplines and locations have contributed to the development of these methods so that a wide range of practical and theoretical strands come together to form the understandings incorporated in this book. Our colleagues include doctors, nurses, social workers, and other health professionals, as well as organizational consultants, management theorists, community psychologists, political activists, liberation theologians, sociodrama practitioners, and community artists. Theoretical understandings either implicit or explicit within the text include those drawn from sociology, anthropology, education, cultural studies, feminism, nursing, family medicine, social work, psychology, post-colonial studies, indigenous knowledges, management, and political science. In all, our text is beholden to an extensive body of work to which many practitioners and theorists have contributed.

While it is impossible to acknowledge all the contributors, particular thanks go to members of our qualitative research study group, Angelita Martini, Roz Walker, Anna Bosco, Rosalie Dwyer, and Jacqui Dodds, who assisted us in clarifying many of the concepts and issues included in this book. We also wish to acknowledge colleagues and fellow travelers Tony Kelly, Susan Young, David Woods, and Jill Abdullah, as well as the staff and students at the Centre for Aboriginal Studies at Curtin University, who have constantly inspired and informed our work. We particularly wish to thank our partners, Rosalie Dwyer and Kathryn Shain, for their insight and wisdom that have contributed so much to our work.

We also wish to thank our editors at Merrill/Prentice Hall, and the reviewers—including Janet M. Boehm, Youngstown State University, and Donald T. Kirkendall, University of North Carolina—whose valuable comments helped us shape and refine the book and make it more accessible to our readers.

Ernie Stringer may be contacted at:
e.stringer@exchange.curtin.edu.au
erniestringer@hotmail.com

Bill Genat may be contacted at:
bgenat@unimelb.edu.au

Brief Contents

1   Action Research for the Health Professions   1

2   Understanding Action Research: Exploring Issues of Paradigm and Method   16

3   Initiating a Study: Research Design   31

4   Gathering Data: Sources of Information   58

5   Giving Voice: Interpretive and Qualitative Data Analysis   89

6   Representation: Communicating Research Processes and Outcomes   115

7   Taking Action: Passion, Purpose, and Pathways   138

8   Action Research in Health: Case Studies   162

9   On-Line Resources   183

References   191

Index   199

Contents

1 Action Research for the Health Professions   1

Action Research in the Health Professions   1
Research Conceptualized   3
Action Research: Systematic Processes of Inquiry   4
Characteristics of Action Research   5
Participatory Processes of Inquiry   9
  Research Roles   10
Working Developmentally: Enlarging the Circle of Inquiry   11
The Changing Health Context   12
Applications of Action Research   13
Summary   15

2 Understanding Action Research: Exploring Issues of Paradigm and Method   16

Introduction   16
Distinguishing Different Approaches to Research: Objective Science and
  Naturalistic Inquiry   16
  Objective Science and Experimental Research   18
  Understanding Human Social Life: Naturalistic Inquiry   20
  Distinguishing Different Types of Evidence   25
Research Relationships in Clinic, Agency, or Community   26
Conclusion   29
Summary   30

3 Initiating a Study: Research Design   31

Setting the Stage: Creating a Productive Research Environment   32
  *With Head, Heart, and Hand: The Human Dimensions of
    Action Research   32*
Research Planning and Design   35
  Building the Researcher's Picture: The Reflective Practitioner   36
  Focusing the Study   37

Framing the Study: Delimiting the Scope of the Inquiry   *39*
Preliminary Literature Review   *40*
Sampling: Selecting Participants   *41*
Sources and Forms of Information (Data Gathering)   *43*
Distilling Information (Analyzing the Data)   *44*
Research Ethics   45
Confidentiality, Care, and Sensitivity   *45*
Permissions   *45*
Institutional Ethical Protocols   *46*
Informed Consent   *46*
Validity in Action Research: A Question of Quality   48
Trustworthiness   *49*
Participatory Validity   *53*
Pragmatic Validity   *53*
An Index of Engagement: Excitement, Interest, Apathy,
   and Resistance   54
Working Principles of Action Research   55
Relationships   *55*
Communication   *56*
Participation   *56*
Conclusion   57
Summary   57

4   Gathering Data: Sources of Information   58

Building a Picture: Gathering Information   59
Interviewing: Guided Conversations   60
Initiating Interviews: Establishing Relationships of Trust   *61*
Questioning Techniques   *62*
Recording Information   *67*
Using Focus Groups to Gather Data   *69*
Overview: Interviews and Focus Groups   *74*
Participant Observation   74
Recording Observations   *75*
Artifacts: Documents, Records, Materials, and Equipment   77
Documents   *78*
Records   *78*
Client Case Notes   *79*
Materials, Equipment, and Facilities   *80*
Recording Information   *81*
Surveys   81
Conducting a Survey   *82*
Statistical and Numerical Data   *83*
Reviewing the Literature   84
Processes for Reviewing/Deconstructing the Literature   *85*
Using the Literature Review   *86*
Developing Insight: Emergent Understandings   87
Summary   88

5 Giving Voice: Interpretive and Qualitative Data Analysis   89

Introduction   90
Data Analysis (1): Analyzing Epiphanies   91
  Epiphanies and Illuminative Experiences   92
  Interpreting Epiphanies and Illuminative Experiences   93
  Selecting Key People   95
  Identifying Epiphanic or Illuminative Experiences   95
  Deconstructing Epiphanies: Features and Elements of Experience   98
  Epiphanies in Observations and Representations   100
  Constructing Conceptual Frameworks   101
  Using People's Terms and Concepts: The Verbatim Principle   102
Data Analysis (2): Categorizing and Coding   103
  Purposes and Processes of Categorizing   103
  Reviewing the Research Question   103
  Reviewing Data Sets   104
  Unitizing the Data   105
  Categorizing and Coding   105
  Organizing a Category System   107
Enhancing Analysis: Incorporating Non-Interview Data   109
Using Category Systems: Frameworks for Reports and Accounts   111
Analyzing Data Collaboratively   111
Conclusion   113
Summary   113

6 Representation: Communicating Research Processes and Outcomes   115

Introduction   116
Communication in Action Research   116
Different Strokes for Different Folks: Forms of Communication   117
Written Reports and Accounts: Writing People's Lives   118
  Life Stories: Biographies, Autobiographies, and Ethnographies   119
  Joint and Collective Accounts: Connecting Stakeholder Experiences   120
  Accumulating Knowledge and Experience   122
  Constructing Reports   123
  Report Formats   126
Presentations: Creative Communication   126
  Audiences and Purposes   127
  Planning Presentations   128
  Enhancing Verbal Presentations: Audio-Visuals   129
  Interactive Presentations   131
Performances: Representing Experience Artistically and Dramatically   132
  Planning Performances: Developing a Script   133
  Producing Performances   134
  Video and Electronic Media   134

Examples of Performances   *135*
Summary   136

7 Taking Action: Passion, Purposes, and Pathways   138

Introduction   139
Engaging People's Passion   140
The Nursing Process and Client Care   141
Assessment   141
Analysis (or Diagnosis)   141
Planning   142
Implementation   142
Evaluation   142
Case Management: Managing Chronic Illness   143
Enhancing Workplace Practices   143
Problem Solving: Action Planning   144
Setting Priorities: Establishing an Action Agenda   145
Creating Pathways: Constructing an Action Plan   145
Reviewing the Plan   146
Supervision: Supporting and Monitoring Progress   147
Evaluation: Assessing the Value and Quality of Programs and Services   148
Everyday Evaluation on the Run   148
Open Inquiry Evaluation   148
Audit Review Evaluation   149
Participatory Evaluation   150
Steps in Collaborative Evaluation   150
Community Development   151
Consensus Building Strategies   152
Empowerment Strategies   153
Developing Health Promotion Programs   154
Professional Development: Collaborative Reflective Practice   156
Strategic Planning: Building the Big Picture   157
Vision Statements   158
Mission Statements   158
Operational Plans   159
Action Plans   159
Summary   160

8 Action Research in Health: Case Studies   162

Introduction   162
1. Self-Care Strategies in Community Nursing   163
2. Psychotherapy: Focusing Client Self-Help Groups   164
3. Health Promotion and Community Development: Hazardous
   Waste Problems   166
4. Creative Prevention Strategies: Hospitals and the Community   167
5. Primary Health Care: Investigating Alcohol Issues   168
6. Parent Participation and Involvement in the Care of a Hospitalized Child   170

7. Change Management in an Interdisciplinary Inpatient Facility within Health Services   172

8. Incorporating the Social Context: Collaborative Reflection within a Family Practice   174

9. Developing Acute Care Protocols in Accident and Emergency   175

10. Integrating the Isolated Aged into Community Practice   176

11. Developing Clinical Protocols for Cataract Surgery   177

12. Action Research and Evidence-Based Wound Management   178

13. Collaborative Inquiry into a WHO Protocol: Stories of Family Physicians   179

14. The Oncology Clinic Tea Trolley: Community Development in Health   180

15. Entry to Cross-Cultural Inquiry: The House Party   181

9   On-Line Resources   183

Introduction   183

On-Line Web Searches   183

Useful Websites   184

General Website Resources   184

Action Research Guidelines and Methodology   185

Women's Health   185

Community Organizations   186

Government-Sponsored Sites   186

Community Health   187

International Organizations   187

Alcohol and Drugs   188

Mental Health   188

Health Promotion   188

HIV   188

University Programs   189

References   191

Index   199

Action Research for the Health Professions

Action Research in the Health Professions

The need for practitioners in the health professions to engage in action research has become increasingly evident. Calls to ground health services in empirical research are matched by demands to demystify health discourses and enable greater participation of both users and providers in the development and evaluation of services (Oliver & Peersman, 2001). Good research, it has been suggested, can elucidate and challenge the status quo and help define future possibilities for concrete action to enhance the day-to-day work of nurses, physicians, therapists, and health promotion and health management professionals as they seek to accomplish the increasingly complex tasks associated with the delivery of effective health care (St Leger & Walsworth-Bell, 1999). Modern health practice expects individual practitioners to develop patient-focused, accessible, evidence-based services in diverse organizational settings. All this occurs in a context where the shifting boundaries between and within the medical, nursing, and allied professions demand the need for practitioners to demonstrate their capacity as knowledgeable actors as they meet service delivery needs and empower their patients (Wicks, 1998; Williams, 2000).

The systematic processes of inquiry available through action research extend the professional capacities of health practitioners, providing methods that improve the effectiveness of interventions and augment professional practice in ways that enhance outcomes for clients. The increasing diversity of modern societies demands the development of appropriate care plans and strategies that fit a client's particular circumstances. Further, the increasing devolution of care requires innovative approaches that enable clients to live well in the community with illness and disability. These circumstances often entail the need for health professionals to engage community or consumer groups in programs and services to foster healthy environments and behaviors (Lupton, Peckham, & Taylor, 1998; Moon, Gould, and Colleagues, 2000; Spencer, Unsworth, & Burke 2001).

Health professionals have used action research to enhance the effectiveness of their work in many different contexts. These include projects that assist clients in developing care plans to improve their health outcomes; that enable clients to forge new ways of living with chronic illness; that assist community and consumer groups to address public health problems; and that set benchmarks of organizational practice for quality assurance in service delivery. The following examples provide a sample of potential applications for action research:

- Tina Koch and Debbie Kralik describe how specialist clinical nurse consultants within their district nursing service investigated incontinence management amongst clients living with multiple sclerosis (Koch, Kralich, Eastwood, & Schofield, 2001; Koch, Kralik, & Kelly, 2000). They assisted a group of women to investigate their incontinence management processes, identify key features of their experience, and formulate action directed toward improving their quality of life. They were able to assist clients to implement, review, and refine alternative strategies that improved the management of incontinence and enhanced their quality of life. At the social level, they successfully petitioned local government for better access to public toilet facilities and had suppliers of containment products improve the delivery systems of their products.
- In his community medical practice, Dr. Ray McKenzie was concerned about the self-care of clients with renal disease. As a part of each consultation, Dr. McKenzie informally inquired about the client's lifestyle. He augmented this inquiry with observations undertaken during home visits and discussions with family members. By collaborating with his clients, Dr. McKenzie was able to take steps to improve the quality of their lives, improve effective service delivery within his own organization, and enhance his own professional practice.
- In her work as a psychotherapist, Jacqui Dodds (1997) was both intrigued and concerned about cancer patients who utilized alternative healing strategies that differed from the biomedical treatments advocated by oncologists. By looking into the experience of other people living with cancer, and through reflection on commonalities and differences, the participants in Dodd's study were able to act in new ways towards their illness. With the support of their fellow participants, they were able to examine and reflect on the outcomes of these actions.
- The manager of a health service in a small town engaged a public health consultant to research problems associated with alcohol use within the local community. Subsequently, research participants identified overzealous policing and the neglect of children as major issues and developed strategies and actions to deal with them.
- Community health workers in an urban health service were interested in examining components of their practice to develop benchmarks, or protocols, with which to guide their practice. They wished to ensure the quality of their practice by using the benchmarks as part of an orientation for new employees. For a year, the health workers met every two weeks to explore key components of their practice—encouraging medication self-management by clients, home visits, administration of client medication records, liaison with the transport section, coordination of client care, development of a care plan, and an overall policy of service delivery. By sharing and analyzing stories of their work, health workers were able to formulate strategies unique to their situation with the frail aged and disabled people who comprised their client group, and to make policy-making recommendations to their organization.

Research Conceptualized

The Merriam-Webster online dictionary (2001) provides the following common ways of using the term "research":

1. The collecting of information about a particular subject
2. Careful or diligent search
3. Studious inquiry or examination
4. Investigation or experimentation aimed at the discovery and interpretation of facts
5. Revision of accepted theories or laws in the light of new facts
6. Practical application of such new or revised theories or laws

Thus, when people research a particular topic related to health services, often they are doing so in the terms indicated by definition 1, collecting information in a general sense. Traditionally, research engaged by scientists and scholars tended to be that related to definitions 4 and 5, though in recent times a broader use includes a more general sense of systematic inquiry implied by definitions 2 and 3. When practitioners engage in *action* research, however, they add another dimension to the definition. They engage in careful, diligent inquiry, not for purposes of discovering new facts or revising accepted laws or theories, but to acquire information having practical application to the solution of specific problems related to their work. This book focuses on the latter use of the term, though its intent is to demonstrate how some of the tools of scientists and scholars may assist professionals in solving significant problems and enhancing their health practices.

The deeper purpose of research is to provide people with knowledge and understanding that makes a difference in their lives. Research is a form of transformational learning that increases the "stock of knowledge" that provides people with the means to engage their lives more effectively. This does not necessarily mean fundamental changes in world view or cultural orientation, though it may, but includes the small "ah-ha's" that enable people to see themselves, others, events, and phenomena with greater clarity or in a positively different way.

Transformational understandings derived from research can provide people with new concepts, ideas, explanations, or interpretations that enable them to see the world in a new way and therefore do things in a different, hopefully better, way. Though any type of learning may provide people with feelings of satisfaction, research provides the possibility of understandings that truly move them into a different universe—the effect of a truly "ah-haaa!" experience, or the "light bulb went on." Good research, for us, is a truly epiphanic experience. We have seen the excitement and delight in people's eyes, heard the wonder in their voices, felt the excitement and sometimes awe that comes with a new way of seeing, and sometimes, a new way of being.

Research, more formally, may be defined as a process of systematic investigation leading to increased understanding of a phenomenon or issue of interest. Though research is ultimately quite an ordinary activity, a process for looking again at an existing situation (researching it), systematic processes of investigation provide the means for ensuring strong and effective processes of inquiry.

Within the academic and professional worlds, two major systems of inquiry—paradigms—provide distinctly different ways in which to investigate phenomena in the physical and human universe. **Objective science**, or **scientific positivism** as it is more correctly known, and **naturalistic inquiry**—often referred to as **qualitative research**—provide powerful but different approaches to research. For purposes of clarity, Chapter 2 explores the nature of the differences between the two paradigms to provide researchers with clearer understandings about the nature of investigations in their own clinics, programs, and services. As the following sections indicate, action research has a history and tradition that differs significantly from other forms of research that have been commonly used to investigate health issues.

Action Research: Systematic Processes of Inquiry

Action research is a systematic, participatory approach to inquiry that enables people to extend their understanding of problems or issues and to formulate actions directed towards the resolution of those problems or issues. Unlike basic research that seeks to formulate explanations that are generalizable to a wide range of contexts within a given population, action research seeks local understandings that are specifically relevant to the particular context of a study.

Although action research has much in common with the regular problem-solving and planning routines used by health practitioners in their daily work in clinic and community, its strength lies in the systematic execution of carefully articulated processes of inquiry. As action researchers they:

- **Design the study,** carefully refining the issue to be investigated, defining the research question, planning systematic processes of inquiry, and checking the ethics and validity of their work
- **Gather data,** including information from a variety of sources
- **Analyze the data** to identify key features of the investigated issue
- **Communicate** the outcomes of the study to relevant audiences
- **Take action** to resolve the investigated issue

Action research usually is cyclical in nature since research participants continuously cycle through processes of investigation as they work towards effective solutions to their research problem. The cycle is often depicted as illustrated in Figure 1.1.

In some contexts, action research is presented as a spiral helix (Figure 1.2) to indicate that phases of the research are repeated over time. Participants in the first instance "Look" at the problem to clarify the nature of the problem, "Think" or reflect on its significance and who is affected by the problem, then "Act" by deciding what action to take. In the next phase, they "Look" again (review) at the actions they have taken, "Think" about those actions to evaluate their effectiveness, then "Act" by extending or refining their actions. The cyclical process continues until an effective solution to the problem has been attained.

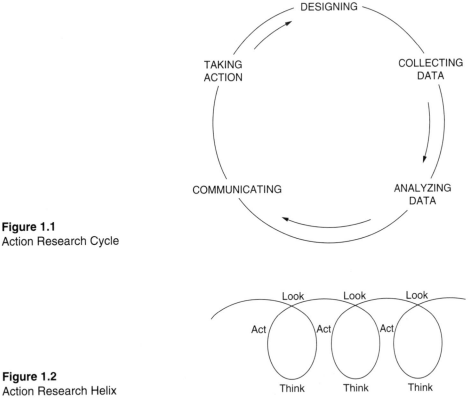

Figure 1.1
Action Research Cycle

Figure 1.2
Action Research Helix

A more complex model of action research is sometimes required for those working in university or professional environments (Figure 1.3). It provides a more detailed profile of the type of activities people engage as they systematically investigate practical problems related to services and practices in their work. The model also indicates how action research differs from objective and generalizable experimental and survey studies that comprise basic epidemiological research. As with other models of action research, it is meant to be a cyclical, reiterative process but is presented in linear form for purposes of clarity.

Characteristics of Action Research

Action research has a long history, one often associated with the work of Kurt Lewin who viewed action research as a cyclical, dynamic, and collaborative process in which people addressed social issues affecting their lives. Through cycles of planning, acting, observing, and reflecting, participants sought changes in practices leading to social action for improvement. A form of action research was used to address problems of assimilation, segregation, and discrimination, to assist people in resolving issues,

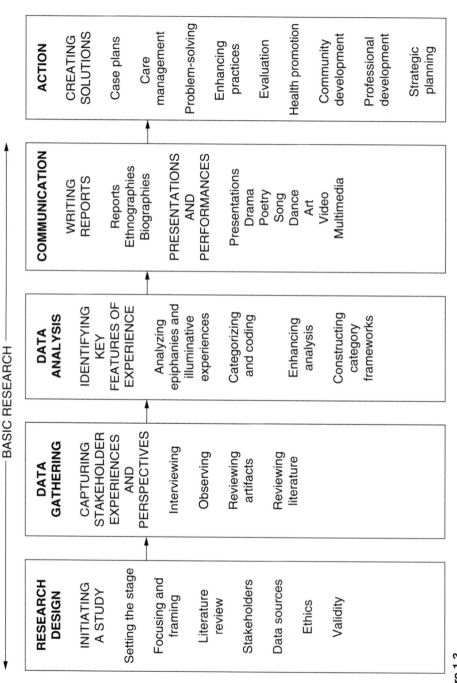

Figure 1.3
Action Research Sequence

6

and to initiate change and study the impact of those changes (Lewin, 1938; Lewin, 1946; Lewin, 1948; Lewin & Lewin, 1942). His approach to action research is reflected in the definition given by Bogdan and Biklen (1992), "the systematic collection of information that is designed to bring about social change."

Kemmis and McTaggart (1988) suggest action research is: "a form of collective, self-reflective enquiry undertaken by participants in social situations in order to improve the rationality and justice of their own social or educational practices, as well as their understanding of these practices and the situations in which these practices are carried out." For Kemmis and McTaggart, research is carried out by any group with a shared concern and is only action research when it is collaborative.

Reason and Bradbury (2002) extend this vision by describing action research as "a participatory, democratic process concerned with developing practical knowing in the pursuit of worthwhile human purposes, grounded in a participatory worldview which we believe is emerging at this historical moment. It seeks to bring together action and reflection, theory and practice, in participation with others, in the pursuit of practical solutions to issues of pressing concern to people, and more generally the flourishing of individual persons and their communities." For them, action research requires skills and methods to enable researchers to foster an inquiring approach to their own practices, to engage in face-to-face work with others to address issues of mutual concern, and to create a wider community of inquiry involving whole organizations.

The need for approaches to research that enable nurses, physicians, and other health professionals to formulate appropriate service delivery practices, and the increasing emphasis on understanding the way lay people may contribute to the development of appropriate health strategies has extended the use of practioner-friendly research methodologies (Abbott & Sapsford, 1997; Fuller & Petch, 1995; Spencer, Unsworth, & Burke, 2001; Taylor, 2000). Stringer (1999) provides a simple Look-Think-Act model that has been applied by health practitioners in a range of community and organizational contexts. More general texts on action research include Berge and Ve (2000); Bray, Lee, Smith, and Yorks (2000); Carr and Kemmis (1986); Carson and Sumara (1997); Coughlan and Brannick (2001); Fals-Borda and Rahman (1991); Heron (1996); McNiff (1995); McNiff, Lomax, and Whitehead (1996); McTaggart (1997); and Schmuck (1997). *The Handbook of Action Research* (Reason & Bradbury, 2001) provides an excellent resource for those engaging in an in-depth study of the theory, principles, and practices of action research.

Not all adherents see action research as necessarily participatory, and there is continuing debate about what counts as action research. In education, Susan Noffke (1997) suggests, "action research is best thought of as a large family, one in which beliefs and relationships vary greatly. More than a set of discrete practices, it is a group of ideas emergent in various contexts. It takes only brief perusal of the action research literature to recognize that the growth and salience of work in this area in recent years have been marked not only by an increase in volume of references but also a proliferation of varied usages of the term" (p. 306). Noffke quotes a generic definition of action research as "research designed to yield practical results that are immediately applicable to a specific situation or problem."

The following section, therefore, provides a description of the features of the approach to action research presented in this book. It differs from much of the literature on practitioner research in that it does not focus solely on practitioner knowledge, though that is an important ingredient. Neither is its primary intent to add to the stock of knowledge available to health practitioners, though the outcomes of action research projects may indeed act in that way. The action research described herein focuses on:

1. **Change:** Improving practices and behaviors by changing them
2. **Reflection:** People thinking, reflecting, and/or theorizing about their own practices, behaviors, and situations
3. **Participation:** People changing their own practices and behaviors, not those of others
4. **Inclusion:** Starting with the agendas and perspectives of the least powerful, widening the circle to include all those affected by the problem
5. **Sharing:** People sharing their perspectives with others
6. **Understanding:** Achieving clarity of understanding of the different perspectives and experiences of all involved
7. **Repetition:** Repeating cycles of research activity leading toward solution to a problem
8. **Practice:** Testing emerging understandings by using them as the basis for changing practices or constructing new practices
9. **Community:** Working toward the development/building of a learning community

The systematic processes of action research extend professional capacities, providing a set of tools that enhance general health service planning and program development. They enable health practitioners to come to grips with significant problems in clinic and community settings that seem impervious to solutions provided by their regular professional stock of knowledge. They are particularly relevant to work in community contexts, especially those involving cultural diversity or situations of poverty or social disruption.

Case Study: Managing Incontinence

Tina Koch and Debbie Kralik (2001c) report how specialist clinical nurse consultants within their district nursing service investigated incontinence management amongst clients living with multiple sclerosis. They sought a participatory method of inquiry that would complement the scope and focus of their existing task and that would enhance their work and their participants' lives through new understandings of living with illness.

They found that Participatory Action Research (PAR), as described by Stringer (1996), accorded with these requirements, "PAR encourages participants to systematically investigate their problems and issues, formulate experiential accounts of their situations, and to devise plans to deal with the issues identified" (Koch & Kralik, 2001c). They also recognized that the underlying principles of PAR—democratic, participatory processes; an equitable perspective that acknowledges people's worth; liberation, providing freedom from oppressive conditions; and life-enhancing, enabling the expression of human potential—accorded with principles of self-determination and empowerment presented in Primary Health Care literature (UNICEF, 1978; World Health Organization, 1978). These principles provided the foundation for their own evidence-based nursing practice and were congruent with their interpretation of the health promotion role of the community nurse.

Four nurse consultants and eight middle-class women living with multiple sclerosis formed the PAR group to inquire into incontinence, a process facilitated by the Director of Research for the nursing service. While the consultants' research question focused on ways that their clients managed incontinence, they also recognized that the women would have their own research questions. Subsequently, the women requested physiological information on how multiple sclerosis affects bladder function. Participants then investigated each other's experiences concerning containment strategies, managing urinary tract infections, interaction with health professionals, the professional understandings of multiple sclerosis, hospitalization, community services, access to toilets, sexual relationships, and strategies for living well in the context of chronic illness (Koch & Kralik, 2001c).

The women identified common themes within their experience, including their lack of voice in the health system and the code of silence surrounding their condition, particularly concerning incontinence and sexuality. They identified the difficulty of obtaining suitable containment products and the lack of appropriate community facilities for the disabled, particularly accessible toilets. Through their dialogue, they validated each other's experiences, created shared meanings of the illness experience, and legitimated and strengthened their sense of self and identity. Particular difficulties and coping behaviors, previously perceived as peculiar, became "normalized" within the group.

By investigating and identifying common features of their experience, the women were able to take action to improve their quality of life. At the individual level, they were able to implement, review, and refine alternative strategies to maintain this quality of life in relation to such issues as the management of incontinence. At the social level, they successfully petitioned local government for better access to public toilet facilities and containment product suppliers for improved delivery systems.

In summary, the authors observe, "A person living with chronic illness may find him/herself in a nexus of dynamic events that may result in a loss of functioning, financial strain, family distress, personal distress, stigma and threats to former self-images. If health care professionals can understand the process that facilitates people to move towards incorporating chronic illness into their lives, we can make a substantial contribution to enhance their chronic disease self-care management and their lives."

Participatory Processes of Inquiry

The participatory processes encompassed by action research enable health professionals to modify the sometimes-alienating procedures of clinical work and move toward a more inclusive process of inquiry. Action research is an alternative approach to research that not only provides diverse inputs of information (data), but is also more amenable to use with lay audiences—clients, families, or community groups. Participatory action research therefore not only provides the technical means for enacting sound health practices, but also for developing a sense of community and living democracy. A major purpose of participatory approaches to inquiry is to bring people together in a dialogic and productive relationship, enabling the development of a sense of community through the sharing of perspectives, the negotiation of meaning, and the development of collaboratively produced activities, programs, and projects.

These principles should not be interpreted as an idealized, utopian fantasy but as pick and shovel, bread and butter issues that are an ordinary part of clinic and community life. Essentially, action research is a participatory approach to inquiry that produces effective and humanized health practices. The search for harmony, peace, love, and happiness needs to sit alongside the search for technical efficiency to become an integral part of the daily processes of clinic and community life. Good health practice is not just about technical or clinical efficiency, but also about the construction of a healthy lifestyle, a healthy workplace, and a healthy community.

The clear message of a participatory approach to action research is that all stakeholders whose lives are affected by an issue need be incorporated into the search for solutions to that issue. The process of collaboratively working toward that goal not only engages a wide range of expertise, both professional and cultural, but also generates positive working relationships. By including patients, clients, and/or families in the search for solutions to problems, we open the possibility of making use of their wisdom and acknowledging the concrete realities effecting client behaviors and health status. Moreover, by engaging them in processes of inquiry that recognizes their competence and worth, we provide the basis for developing productive relationships engendering trust and understanding. Even the poorest family or community has a store of experience and knowledge that can be incorporated into meaningful activities with the power to attain the health outcomes desired by professionals and their clients.

Research Roles

The time honored roles in research have traditionally been simple to track, comprised of "researchers" (and possibly "associates" and "assistants") who control and implement the research and "subjects" (or sometimes "informants") who are the objects of research. Action research roles are not as easy to define, since people may have multiple roles and sometimes change roles in the course of a study.

Health professionals who engage in research related to their professional practices may be designated "researchers" or "practitioner researchers." When they engage colleagues and clients in participatory research, they may be termed "research facilitators" whose role is to assist these other participants in planning and conducting the research. People may be drawn into the research process as "participants" by providing information (data), but when they contribute to the planning and conduct of the research they may also be termed "researchers." Generally, both researchers and participants are drawn from "stakeholders"—those who have a "stake" in the research because they are affected by the issue at hand (e.g., clients, professionals, care-givers, and so on), or because they have an influence on events related to the issue (administrators, policymakers, funders, and so on).

In the text that follows, those who participate in the research in any capacity will be designated as "participants," and those who are responsible for the conduct of the research—planning, gathering and analyzing data, writing reports, and so on—will be referred to as "researchers." The most powerful action research processes emerge when all participants become researchers in their own right, gaining the skills and insights that enable them to systematically investigate issues in their own lives.

Working Developmentally: Enlarging the Circle of Inquiry

Although action research works effectively for discrete problems and issues within a clinic, it has the potential for more extended applications across organizations or within the community. As participants cycle through a research process, new understandings often reveal critical issues going beyond the immediate focus of investigation that point to productive possibilities that might increase the scope and power of inquiry. Investigation of specific problems often reveals the multiple dimensions of the situation, and investigation of each of those dimensions further illuminates the situation, revealing additional possibilities for action.

The process of starting small and increasing the breadth and complexity of activity is called working developmentally. Though somewhat different from constructs within developmental psychology or child development, there are some conceptual similarities. In each, it is important to engage clients with familiar ideas and concepts, then introduce more complex issues as their understanding develops. A study may start with limited objectives that are extended as understanding and awareness increase. The potential for positive change and development increases exponentially as increasing numbers of people and issues are included (Figure 1.4).

A key feature of the developmental process is to start with limited objectives. Although many problems within health services are complex and multidimensional in scope, it is best to focus initial inquiries on tangible and achievable objectives. Small initial gains provide people with the stimulus of success and inspire them to take further action. By engaging continuous cycles of the "Look-Think-Act" process, they are able

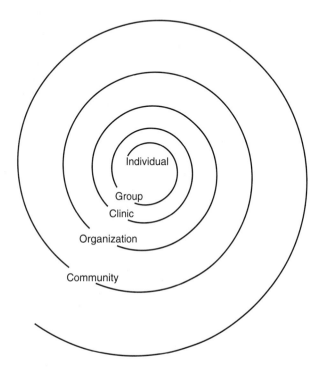

Figure 1.4
Action Research Spiral

to encompass more dimensions of the problem and increased levels of engagement. Eventually, they may be able to incorporate other stakeholders—thus marshalling increased levels of support and resources that extend the power of actions they take.

> Wadsworth (2001) describes a study that commenced with the intention of investigating mental health service user views of a large central city psychiatric hospital. Iterative research cycles incorporated increasingly broad processes of inquiry among staff and consumers of mental health services. "Work with the initial ward extended and expanded upwards, outwards, and iteratively: to all wards in the hospital, then to the Area Mental Health Service, other area services, to the region, and state and finally federal levels of government policy and funding administration" (Wadsworth, 2001, p. 424). The study eventually encompassed activity that enabled research participants to accomplish systematic change in the way consumers participated in mental health service quality improvement.

The Changing Health Context

Action research emerges in a social and professional context that is driven by continuing changes to health policies, programs, and services that require more sophisticated understandings of the nature of health issues. Nurses, physicians, therapists, and allied health professionals draw on a wide range of research traditions to enhance their expertise and attain effective service delivery outcomes. Action research has emerged as an additional tool to apply to their work, providing a practical and rigorous means to enhance expertise and develop practice. While health practices have traditionally focused on biomedical, curative care provided in hospital and clinical settings, health services now encompass a much broader range of activity that includes preventative, curative, and rehabilitative services in clinical, family, and community contexts.

Grounded in biomedical science, Western medicine and health practices have indeed made giant steps in preventing disease and curing common ailments. The continuing extension of biomedical approaches to health, however, is limited by two major factors: the huge expense of maintaining institutionally based health and medical services, and the concomitant realization that sound health care practices must, ultimately, reside in the community—in people's homes and families. At least part of this realization arises because of the difficulties experienced in preventing people from engaging in risky health behaviors—smoking, unsafe sexual practices, poor dietary habits, lack of exercise, and so on—and maintaining treatments and medication schedules for specific illnesses and conditions. Contemporary perspectives on the treatment of the aged and infirm have likewise changed the landscape of health services delivery.

Attempts to come to grips with these issues have spawned significant changes in the way health professionals think about health issues, and in the way governments and health services organize their programs and services. These changes are driven, to some extent, by continuing changes in social and cultural demographics, so that there is continuing pressure, on both pragmatic and political grounds, to ensure that health services are accessible, effective, and appropriate to the populations for which they are designed. Muslim and Jewish dietary prescriptions and proscriptions, for instance, must now be taken into account in settings as diverse as Birmingham, Chicago, and Sydney, and birth control and fertility programs have different connotations in third world and middle-class Western environments. Social and cultural sensitivities, together with broader understandings of public health, have resulted in a variety of changes in health practice. These include:

- **Community care:** The development of integrated, multidisciplinary approaches to community care that provide appropriate and sensitive policies and practices (Bytheway et al., 2001). The development of partnerships in care for both curative and preventative services (Komaromy, 2001) means that family and community nurses can strengthen the levels of care available to patients by working collaboratively with families (Whyte, 1997).
- **Changes to nursing practice:** New ways of thinking about nursing roles at a time when nursing practice is expanding (Allen, 2000) and boundaries between and within the professions of medicine and nursing are shifting (Ross & MacKenzie, 1996; Wicks, 1998; Williams, 2000).
- **Public involvement:** A growing emphasis on public involvement in health care decision making, focusing on the consumer or user of services (Komaromy, 2001; Lupton, Peckham, & Taylor, 1998). This increases in importance as competing paradigms related to such issues as reproduction point to the strong links between the biological and the social (Kent, 2000).
- **The changing status of Western scientific knowledge:** The continued questioning of orthodox scientific views of health and disease, the coexistence of lay beliefs and complementary or alternative therapies, and the place of ritual, relationships of trust, and communication between physicians and patients (Seale, Pattison, & Davey, 2001). These movements are complemented by increasing acceptance of lay knowledge in the development of health care services (Rogers, Hassell, & Nicolaas, 1998). They point to the need to develop alternative epidemiologies that draw on lay knowledge and recognize the contextual factors influencing health status (Moon et al., 2000).

Applications of Action Research

The literature on action research is now voluminous. Though it has become widely used in education, it is now emerging as a significant tool for the health professions. Hart and Bond (1995) provide a guide to research in health and social care that seeks to demystify some of the research thinking processes. Winter and Munn-Giddings (2001) offer a guide to action research as a strategy for inquiry and development in health and social care. Spencer, Unsworth, and Burke (2001) suggest ways community health nurses can develop patient-focused services. Mienczakowski and Morgan (2001) describe how they apply action research with health care patients and professionals to such issues as schizophrenia, drug and alcohol abuse, and sexual assault recovery. Barrett (2001) highlights how action research—informed by feminist processes—was applied within midwifery. Hills (2001) shows how cooperative inquiry, a form of action research, was used to create methods of evaluation that are compatible with the new human science, caring paradigm. Wadsworth (2001) describes how action research was used to facilitate development of mental health services in a large central city psychiatric hospital. Benner (1994) presents another related methodology—interpretive phenomenology—that explores embodiment, caring, and ethics in health care practices. She provides examples of ways this approach to research has been applied to work with teenage mothers (Smithbattle, 1994), schizophrenia within families (Chesla, 1994), care of hospitalized children (Darbyshire, 1994), stroke recovery (Doolittle, 1994), living with chronic illness (Benner, Janson-Bjerklie, Ferketich, & Becker, 1994), dying patients (Wros, 1994), cancer (Gordon, 1994), and disaster recovery (Stuhlmiller, 1994). Van Willigen (1993) provides case studies of ways action anthropology has been applied to health issues in low income and urban contexts.

The literature incorporates diverse orientations that derive from the different theories used by the writers, the assumptions drawn from these theories about what should or could be accomplished, and the set of appropriate practices that are therefore entailed. Noffke (1997), for instance, defines differences in action research according to their personal, professional, and political dimensions. Some authors present a naturalistic approach to research, seeking to engage practitioners in reflective processes illuminating significant features of their professional practice and enabling them to understand the experience and perspective of other participants in clinic and community contexts (Taylor, 2000).

As a tool for practitioners, action research provides the means for health practitioners to enhance their practice by engaging in systematic inquiry with those with whom they work—patients, clients, administrators, colleagues, families, and community groups. Action research can be applied in a broad range of contexts—in hospital, clinic, and community—for the development of any of the following:

- Curative or preventative interventions and practices
- Health and wellness programs
- Coping strategies
- Health assessment
- Program or service evaluation
- Care plans
- Health care systems
- Health care delivery
- Family and community nursing
- Health plans and strategies
- Health promotion plans, strategies, and programs

Action research processes have been successfully applied to a range of issues and conditions, including:

- Chronic conditions
- Stress
- Pregnancy and childbirth
- Medication regimens
- Pain management

- Hygiene
- Sexuality
- Incontinence
- Loss, grieving, and death
- Sleep management
- Nutrition
- Rehabilitation
- Drug and alcohol misuse
- Physical therapy

Through systematic processes of inquiry and development, therefore, action research provides a set of tools to enable health professionals to develop effective practices that achieve positive outcomes for their patients and clients.

SUMMARY

The Purposes of Action Research

Action research is a process of systematic inquiry.

The purpose of action research is to provide health practitioners with new knowledge and understanding enabling them to improve professional practices or resolve significant problems in clinical and community settings.

Action research derives from a research tradition emphasizing dynamic approaches to investigation that are:

- **Reflective**
- **Participatory**
- **Cyclical**
- **Focused on understanding**
- **Change-oriented**
- **Community-oriented**

A common process of inquiry includes:

- **Design of the study**
- **Data gathering**
- **Data analysis**
- **Communicating outcomes**
- **Taking action**

Action research may be engaged as a developmental process that systematically increases the scope of the investigation.

It is a tool of investigation that has application to a wide range of health service delivery issues and problems.

Understanding Action Research: Exploring Issues of Paradigm and Method

Introduction

One of the difficulties of engaging in health research is the proliferation of methods employed. Thirty years ago the term *research* was used in university or professional contexts to refer to scientific research. This term commonly referred to experimental, epidemiological, or *quantitative* research that was seen as the epitome of scientific investigation. The search for "factual" information encompassed by this view of research has been complemented by an understanding that other forms of research entailing different methods of investigation may be useful sources of information. Today a variety of *qualitative* studies also inform the health arena, providing different forms of "evidence" to assist health professionals engage in effective service delivery.

Underlying the different research methodologies is an assumption that different types of knowledge often are needed to accomplish effective health outcomes. To clarify the differences between the research methodologies related to these different forms of knowledge, this chapter will explore the distinctions between the two major paradigms, commonly called quantitative research and qualitative research. The intent is to assist practitioners to understand more clearly when and how different methodologies might appropriately be applied to health issues and problems.

Distinguishing Different Approaches to Research: Objective Science and Naturalistic Inquiry

Systematic research continues to be the source of information that informs the curative and preventative procedures and practices of health professionals. Carefully designed studies continue to extend our understanding of the complex processes involved in fighting sickness and disease and establishing the well-being of people. While epidemiological research plays a predominant role in health-related investigations, today it is widely recognized that other forms of research provide distinctly different ways to provide health practitioners with the knowledge that will make their work more efficient and effective. **Objective science** or **positivism,** often designated as quantitative research, and **naturalistic inquiry,** commonly designated as qualitative research, provide powerful but different approaches to research that have applications in health.

In general terms, research promises to assist health practitioners by providing scientifically validated knowledge, or by providing the means to find workable solutions to problems they confront in their day-to-day work. There are times when they need to observe the situation objectively and to develop appropriate diagnoses and treatments of a client's "condition," irrespective of what the client may think or feel. At these times, they engage the standpoint of objective science, seeking to establish the facts of the situation and to apply scientifically formulated explanations to the problem at hand.

At other times, however, these procedures will prove inadequate, the nature of the problem being deeply integrated with social and cultural issues that are not readily amenable to detached scientific techniques and procedures. In these circumstances, **qualitative** or **naturalistic** approaches to research provide a different set of tools to deal with the situation. They provide the means to investigate the social and cultural complexities within which the health problem is enmeshed. In particular, they offer greater insight into the ways people interpret events from their own perspective, providing culturally and contextually appropriate information assisting practitioners to more effectively manage problems they and their clients confront.

Many health professionals continue to be frustrated by clients who continue to engage in health-threatening and, in some cases, life-threatening behaviors. Inappropriate diets, alcohol, cigarettes, lack of exercise, and so on continue to plague the populations of so-called "advanced" nations. These cases are mirrored in developing nations, where people continue to engage in high-risk behaviors because they are seen as culturally appropriate. Often, the scientific knowledge is not heeded because it requires changes in long-standing cultural practices and habits.

Many of our colleagues express continuing frustration at their inability to convince patients of the need for particular dietary or care regimes. I am not immune from this myself, as I know from my experience of a recent rehabilitation for a skiing injury. Although I was told of the reasons for the required exercises, I found it difficult to fit them into my daily routine, and the shoulder did not heal as quickly as it otherwise might have. The scientific knowledge related to the mechanics of my body needed to be supplemented by an exploration of my everyday life. Only by putting those two forms of knowledge together could I accomplish the rehabilitation of my shoulder.

Health professionals therefore need to keep in mind the essential differences between positivistic and naturalistic approaches to research—the former is more intent on precise measurements that produce objective knowledge, and the latter is more focused on the subjective construction of meaning that extends our understanding of people's life experiences. The distinction has implications for different ways of responding to health issues and problems—positivism that seeks quantifiable measurements that point to the best solution to a problem, and naturalistic inquiry that is more focused on ways of constructing solutions to problems that are grounded in cultural meanings.[1]

Objective Science and Experimental Research

One of the enduring legacies of the modern world is that bestowed by science. So successful has science been at providing miraculous material benefits to human life that scientific knowledge has achieved a preeminent status that puts it above all others. In recent decades, billions of dollars have been invested in scientific health and medical research, providing a huge body of knowledge that has effectively been applied to both curative and preventative practices, services, and programs.

This body of "scientific" knowledge derived from a philosophical perspective is technically known as scientific positivism. Scientific positivism operates according to a particular set of underlying assumptions and beliefs about the way knowledge can be acquired. It assumes a fixed universe that operates according to a stable set of laws defining the phenomena and the relationship between those phenomena. Positivism assumes that ultimately, in principal, everything in the universe can be measured with precision, and the relationship between phenomena described accurately. Continuing scientific efforts to refine and extend our understanding of the universe are carried out in the disciplinary spheres of physics, chemistry, biology, and so on. Each has a distinctive focus, providing scientifically verified information extending our understanding of the physical universe. Physiology and human biology focus on those aspects of the universe dealing with the human body, but generally stop short of involvement of the mind, that aspect of the universe that is peculiar to human beings.

The purpose of scientific inquiry, therefore, is to describe with precision the features of the universe and the stable relationships that hold between those features. Scientific work is often associated with accurate definition and measurement of variables to determine the nature and extent of those relationships, the ultimate goal being to establish causal connections (e.g., the effect of a particular chemical on the operation of a particular aspect of the human body; the impact of a particular intervention on health-related behaviors; and so on). The success of science in establishing those stable sets of relationships has enabled the production of the technological marvels of the modern world—a huge array of medications for treating many conditions; manufactured materials to substitute for parts of the natural human body; surgical processes for altering or repairing the functioning of the human body; the curing of illness; and the eradication of diseases.

Once science is able to measure and describe precisely the nature of a particular set of phenomena, it is able to predict how those phenomena behave with a great

---

[1] We need to be wary of interpreting this simplistically, since good professionals probably incorporate both elements into their practice.

deal of certainty. Scientific investigation, with its emphasis on precise measurement and careful analysis, provides the basis for explanations of the working of the human body. The outcome of the application of scientific principles to the development of explanation and understanding is a highly sophisticated and rigorous stock of scientific knowledge resulting in many advances in health policies, practices, and technologies. The knowledge emerging from positivistic science continues to have the potential to dramatically enhance people's lives.

This has obvious implications for health services and practices. If health professionals can scientifically measure and describe the precise nature of problems people experience, then they should, in theory, be able to control all of the factors likely to influence a client's well-being and therefore produce highly effective outcomes for each and every person. Armed with scientific knowledge, they should be able to predict with precision the conditions required for any person to acquire the information necessary to achieve a healthy life, irrespective of his/her gender, class, ethnicity, or any other factor likely to affect their well-being.

The primary method for establishing scientific explanations is the experimental method. The purpose of experiments is to provide the means for establishing cause-effect relationships between phenomena. Experimental studies try to establish the causes and effects of different illnesses or conditions and the effects of interventions and plans. This enables professional practitioners to explain the factors causing problems and to predict the conditions that will alleviate them. Experiments are carefully constructed to ensure that plausible rival explanations may account for phenomena observed.

Quasi-experiments, or non-experiments as they are sometimes called (Johnson, 2001), are used where it is not possible to manipulate variables experimentally, either for ethical or pragmatic reasons. It would be difficult to imagine setting up a study in which participants were exposed to major health risks with no certainty of effective intervention. What is possible, in these situations, is to engage in studies where variables are controlled or manipulated statistically rather than experimentally, establishing the nature of the relationship between variables by carefully contrived statistical manipulation. Epidemiological researchers are able to employ statistical methods that control for a wide range of variables and, in the process, minimize the plausibility of rival explanations for the effects observed.

Both experimental and quasi-experimental research is subject to forms of quality control to ensure rigor in procedure and stability of results. For these reasons, experiments are evaluated according to their reliability, internal validity, and external validity—the extent to which similar results may be obtained from different settings, samples, and times (reliability); the extent to which results might be attributed to the experimental variables (internal validity); and the extent to which results apply to the broader population from which the sample was drawn (external validity or generalizability).

Experimental and quasi-experimental research has provided a large array of information having the potential to dramatically improve people's social health and well-being. As will become evident in the following discussion, however, health problems continue to proliferate, despite the huge array of scientifically validated knowledge now at our disposal. Although scientific positivism has provided a powerful body of knowledge about the operation of the human body and the nature of the physical environment, understanding human social and cultural contexts has proven much more elusive, and other research strategies have emerged enabling different ways of understanding these issues and problems.

Understanding Human Social Life: Naturalistic Inquiry

The problem with applying science to human affairs lies in the nature of humanity. We are at once physical, biological, and socio-cultural beings, and attempts to understand our behavior need to take into account each of those facets. While the methods of positivistic science are powerful ways of understanding our physical being and provide deep insights into our biological nature, they come up short as vehicles for providing explanations for the socio-cultural aspects of human life. Although experimentation still assists us to understand certain features of human social and cultural life, ultimately positivistic explanations must fail to encompass some of the fundamental features of human life—the creative and willful construction of meaning that is at the center of every social activity. It is the need to investigate meaning that is at the heart of naturalistic inquiry.

While experimental science has provided much useful information about the physical aspects of health, any theory of human behavior can only be a tentative, partial explanation of any individual or group's acts or behaviors. Two things intervene in attempts to describe scientific laws of human behavior. One is the nature of human beings themselves. As cross-cultural studies have demonstrated convincingly, people perceive the world and respond to it in many different ways. Given the same sets of facts, people will interpret both what they are seeing and what that means differently. No amount of explanation or clarification can provide a set of foundational truths about the way people should behave, since behavior is predicated on sets of beliefs that are not, in principle, verifiable. Any "truth" of human experience is true only within a given framework of meanings.

This becomes increasingly clear if we consider some of the fundamental conditions of human social life and the way they impact the lives of individuals. The concept of the life-world comes to us from the work of sociologists like Peter Berger (Berger & Luckman, 1967; Berger, Berger, & Kellner, 1973) who engage research from the perspective that people construct reality as an ongoing social process in their everyday lives. The life-world refers to the consciousness of everyday life that is carried by every individual and provides coherence and order to their existence. The life-world is not a genetically inherited view of the world, but is learned by individuals as they experience everyday events and interactions within the compass of their families and communities. The life-world is therefore socially constructed, so that individuals learn to live in a social world according to sets of meaning deeply embedded in their everyday conduct and shared by others living in that particular place and time.

The life-world is not a random set of events, but is given order and coherence by a patterned, structured organization of meaning that is so ordinary that people literally do not see it. People are usually not conscious of the depth and complexity of the worlds they inhabit. A child learns to associate with parents and siblings in particular ways, to communicate using a particular language, to act in particular ways, to participate in events like meals, conversation, play, work, and so on, using appropriate behaviors and routine ways of accomplishing his/her everyday life. Like a fish in the sea, people cannot see the "water" of this patterned, structured everyday life, but live in a taken-for-granted social world providing order and coherence for all aspects of their everyday lives—the interactions, acts, activities, events, purposes, feelings, and productions that comprise their lives.

> We get some idea of what this means when we visit a new place for the first time, especially if it is in a foreign country. We feel uncomfortable to varying degrees until we learn the "rules" that enable us to operate in the new setting—the appropriate words to use, how to sit or stand, how to eat, how to dress appropriately, and so on. We become aware of a myriad of small behaviors that those living in the context take for granted because it is so much an ordinary part of their life-world.
>
> I remember people's consternation when I visited an Indigenous community for the first time and sat with my wife in church, not realizing that the sexes had been strictly segregated and that I was sitting with the women. I've also inadvertently entered a female restroom and felt embarrassed by the surprised exclamations of the women there and my flustered retreat. Small and apparently inconsequential behaviors can sometimes have quite a dramatic impact on our ability to interact comfortably with people.

The anthropologist Goodenough (1971) conceptualized this life-world in terms of the concept culture, which he defined as the socially learned rules and boundaries that enable a person to know what *is* (how the world is *defined*, structured, made up), what *can be* (what is *possible* in the world, whether it be ancestral ghosts, the existence of God, or faster than light travel), what *should be* (the system of values enabling the individual to distinguish between good and bad, appropriate and inappropriate), *what to do* (what acts or behaviors are required to accomplish a purpose) and *how to do it* (the steps required to accomplish that purpose). Individuals, therefore, inhabit a life-world comprised of taken-for-granted rules and boundaries giving order and coherence to their lives. Without these patterns and structures of meaning, people would live in a bewildering, chaotic world of sensation and events that would make human life as we know it impossible. It is this cultural cradle that enables us to live together in harmony, to accomplish day-to-day tasks like eating meals, dressing, communicating through talk and discussion, working, resolving disputes, and mowing the lawn.

Though we live within a particular life-world made of sets of meaning deeply embedded in our life histories, we are usually not conscious of the rules, boundaries, routines, or recipes giving meaning and coherence to our lives. The taken-for-granted world is not seen, or apprehended, but *lived*. Recent anthropological explorations, therefore, focus on the primacy of experience (Bruner, 1986; Jackson 1996), using Dilthey's (1976) notion that reality exists only in the facts of consciousness given by inner experience. We can understand the social world, however, only through apprehending the cultural texts (Barthes, 1986; Ricoeur, 1979) or discourses through which people communicate their experience. Often, we become aware of the personal/shared nature of our taken-for-granted world when we come in conflict with another discourse—when disjuncture occurs in our interactions with others.

The distinctive aspect of our cultural life-world, therefore, is that we share it with people who have learned similar sets of meanings and who act according to the patterns and structures of meaning with those who have had similar life experiences. But beneath the apparent order and coherence of the social life-world is a deeply chaotic system of meanings that continually threatens the possibility of an ordered and productive daily life. For each person has had somewhat different experiences, and each has built a system of meanings that works superficially to accomplish ordinary tasks, but has slightly different nuances and interpretations. At any one time these differences can be magnified and distorted, causing confusion or conflict as people try to accomplish their everyday lives. This is readily apparent when people get married and discover that a person with whom they thought they shared deeply consonant views of the world evinces acts and behaviors not in accord with their own. Small acts—the dropping of a sock or tissue, the use of a word—can trigger discomfort, discordance, and even conflict. The art of marriage requires people to learn new sets of meaning and to negotiate acts and behaviors consonant with a partner's existing habits and values in order to accomplish a life together. It is something that is sometimes astonishingly difficult, even for people closely committed to each other.

This discordance of perspectives is particularly relevant in health-related contexts. Toombs (1993) reveals, "In discussing my illness with physicians, it has often seemed to me that we have been somehow talking at cross-purposes, discussing different things, never quite reaching one another." These cross-purposes arise, she suggests, not from insensitivity or inattentiveness, but from a fundamental disagreement about the nature of illness, so that health professionals constantly confront clients whose realities appear to fly in the face of concrete evidence that lies before their very eyes.

One of the major tasks of qualitative research, therefore, is to uncover the meanings implicit in the acts and behaviors of interacting individuals. By exploring the world of others, we seek to understand what they experience and the meaning given to that experience. In other words, through an increased understanding of people's divergent life-worlds we seek ways of redoing, reenacting, and/or reconceptualizing events in ways that will make sense to all people involved.

This is not just a technical task, but involves deeply held feelings associated with the meanings implicit in a person's life-world. Not only are people attached to their particular life-worlds emotionally, they also react unfavorably when it is threatened. A denial of the veracity or validity of any aspect of a person's life-world is likely to create negative feelings that inhibit the possibility of productive interaction. The world of human life is meaningful, interactional, emotional, and constructive, and accomplishing productive and harmonious human activity requires all these aspects of experience to be taken into account. It is this understanding that is at the heart of action research—the need to clarify and understand the meaning implicit in the acts and behaviors of all people involved in events on which research is focused, and the need to use those extended understandings as the basis for resolving the problems investigated.

This lesson is deeply inscribed in my consciousness. As a young teacher, I worked with the children of Australian Aboriginal people who lived a very traditional hunter-gatherer lifestyle. It soon became evident to me that they literally lived in a different universe—that the way they viewed the world, the way they acted towards each other, and their aspirations and responses were so dramatically different from my own that my teaching made absolutely no sense to their everyday world. I became aware of the need to come to know something of that world in order to provide a bridge of understanding between their world and the curriculum that I was teaching.

Even the simplest aspects of the syllabus entailed elements that were deeply engaged with the different visions of the world and the lifestyles attached. As I watched the people engaged in the simple act of gathering seeds and fruit from the plants in the desert to provide for their immediate needs, I became aware of how deeply embedded I was in the world of technological production when I cut a slice of bread for my lunch. Behind that simple act lay the mining and production of metals needed for the knife, as well as that required for the production of the machinery needed to grow and process the wheat, and to fabricate the ovens and other machinery needed to make the bread. What I had seen as a simple loaf of bread became a complex technological production.

My eyes began to see a different world when I asked the question, "What do I need to know in order to understand where this bread came from?" A very different order of understanding came to mind when I asked, "What do Aboriginal people need to know when they ask a similar question about their own foodstuffs?" Not only does the actual world of technological production intrude, but the web of work and economic relationships enabling me to acquire that loaf of bread are likewise complex and very different from the web of relationships surrounding Aboriginal meals.

This experience changed forever the way I interact with other people, including my circle of friends. I now realize the need to find ways of making connections between what others know—how they perceive and understand the world from the standpoint of their own history of experience—and what I need to know to interact with them harmoniously and successfully. That fundamental perception has been recently reinforced as I've worked in the United States where the experiences and perspectives of Hispanic and African American people have enriched and challenged my educational endeavors. As I worked in the South Valley in Albuquerque and the poorer suburbs of Columbia and Richmond, I had much learning to do before I could frame my knowledge in ways that made sense to people in those places. The same dynamic operated in my work with youth in London, where I had to engage in some on-the-spot research to enable me to work effectively.

Differences in cultural perspective do not relate to ethnic differences alone, however. We have only to look at the differences in the way teenagers and their parents interpret events to realize the extent to which age differentials create differences in cultural experience and perspective in everyday life. Parents listening to their children's music often shake their heads in wonder that *anyone* could find the experience pleasurable, a response mirrored by teenagers listening to their parents' music. They all are hearing the same music, in terms of the sounds emanating from the instrument or recording, but they have very different experiences of the sounds and associate very different meanings with them.

The perspectives from sociology and anthropology presented in the previous section are clearly associated with phenomenology, a philosophical standpoint that explores the subjective dimensions of human experience. Phenomenology focuses on the need to get subjectively in touch with knowledge of people's everyday experience, not so that we can *explain* it through our own systems of knowledge, but so that we can understand it in their terms.

The implications for health practitioners are clear. Phenomenology does not offer theory to explain and/or control practitioner/client interactions and behaviors, but rather offers plausible insights that have the potential to connect health professionals more meaningfully with the world of their clients and patients. Benner (1994) suggests that "caring, as a way of helping people by entering their world, is a higher kind of knowledge, which we can call understanding and the potential of . . . practical wisdom." She further proposes that "experts in caring know they cannot be guided by principles or any pseudo-sciences of the psyche, but must enter into the situation of the patient. . . ." This does not mean that science does not have a place in caring. As Benner points out (1994), only by combining technological and existential skills can we approach healing the embodied person.

A phenomenological perspective should not be interpreted as *the* best way to approach research, since it will sometimes be appropriate for practitioners and researchers to stand back and observe the situation objectively, assessing and evaluating events in unemotional and disengaged terms. At other times, however, they need to enter the life-world of their clients to understand how to construct processes or practices that "make sense" within their everyday lives. The processes of action research provide the means to transact these apparently incommensurable, incompatible "stocks-of-knowledge," enabling people to collaboratively and interactively seek ways of understanding that "make sense" to all involved.

Action research, therefore, employs interpretive processes of qualitative inquiry as a central dynamic of investigation. Its purpose is to commence inquiry by describing and giving meaning to events, . . . showing how they are perceived and interpreted by actors in the setting. By studying events in this way, we are able to better understand or comprehend people's experience. Taking an interpretive approach to qualitative research, action research therefore:

- Identifies different definitions of the problem
- Reveals the perspectives of the various interested parties

- Suggests alternative points of view from which the problem can be interpreted and assessed
- Identifies strategic points of intervention
- Exposes the limits of statistical information by furnishing materials that enable the understanding of individual experiences

Qualitative, interpretive approaches to inquiry, therefore, provide the principle means for enabling health practitioners to engage action research to devise strategies more attuned to the realities of people's lives. While it is useful in some contexts to think of them in objective terms, to plan strategies and interventions that enable effective outcomes, there will be times when the collaborative construction of care processes or the formulation of socially and culturally appropriate programs will be enhanced by the processes explored in the coming chapters.

When I first entered university life, I was the sole arbiter of the content and processes of teaching in my courses. I formulated the syllabus from the content of my professional expertise and ensured that I maintained carefully controlled instructional processes in order to ensure that students in my class learned systematically.

As a result of my experiences in many different cultural contexts, my preparation for classes and my teaching is much more flexible and participatory. I engage my students in the process of assisting me to formulate a syllabus and, in the process, try to accommodate the diverse backgrounds and learning styles with which they come to my classes. That doesn't mean that I do not prepare thoroughly, or that classroom management is never an issue, but preparation and management have necessarily become a collaborative process.

At first, as I learned how to do this, it seemed like extra work, but having become more skilled, I can now accomplish it easily. Further, I've learned that by engaging students in these processes they not only become more interested and enthusiastic about their learning, but also have some wonderful ideas about both the content and the processes of learning.

While I still appreciate and make use of the information acquired from my studies of psychology, sociology, and anthropology—much of it gained through experimental or quasi-experimental research—I am able to place that alongside the knowledge I acquire of my students' experience using naturalistic techniques of inquiry. Each has its place. Each provides tools for acquiring knowledge.

Distinguishing Different Types of Evidence

As practitioners read research reports and formulate evaluative activities related to their ongoing work, they will need to clearly distinguish between the different types of information presented or required. They will be confronted with a variety of different types of information, some of it derived from experimental studies based on fixed measurements of carefully defined variables, or descriptive information related to the socio-cultural and interactive dimensions of people's experience. Information will be acquired by different means, and be used for different purposes, providing an array of knowledge that will be relevant to different aspects of professional practice. Practitioners will need to be clear about the type of information they require and to make judgments about the way it might best be used.

Research Relationships in Clinic, Agency, or Community

The changes in methods signaled by the move from experimental to qualitative research, however, also reflect a change in the human dimensions of investigation. Whereas experimental research starts from the assumption that the researcher takes a disinterested, objective view in order to acquire unbiased, objective truths, action research assumes an engaged and subjective interaction with people in the research setting.

There are, however, deeper issues to be considered in engaging participatory action research as a mode of inquiry. Modern social life, with its tendency toward centralized bureaucratic forms of organization, too easily slides into a form of autocratic operation at odds with the democratic intent of its institutions. Too often, powerful figures in professional contexts take on the manner and style of an authority, imposing their perspectives and agendas on others and disregarding their needs and views. Though this sometimes works—the authority-figure director who keeps an iron hand on the reins of the agency; or the demanding, disciplinary administrator who will not countenance poor behavior or performance—it provides a poor model of life in a democratic society. Too often, people accept the unacceptable and are passive contributors to processes that inhibit or sometimes damage their lives or the lives of their children.

The import of this issue, broadly speaking, is that a set of **relationships** has been built into professional life that sometimes needs to be modified in order to carry out an effective action research process. A common assumption built into interactions between professionals and their client groups says, in effect, "I'm the expert here. I know what needs to be done." The assumption here is that training and experience have provided professionals with special knowledge enabling them to make definitive judgments about the nature of the problem experienced and to formulate appropriate solutions to the problem. While this works in some instances, or in instances where the clients are culturally and socially similar to the professional, there are many instances where the "expert" knowledge of the professional does not provide the basis for an effective solution to the problem. Some of the deep-seated and long-standing problems in human services relate to the imposition of Eurocentric, middle-class-oriented systems of understanding being imposed onto people—clients, community groups, and sometimes fellow professionals—whose social and cultural orientations are quite different.

Interpretive action research, therefore, starts from quite a different position. It says, in effect, "Although I have professional knowledge that may be useful in exploring the issue or problem facing us, my knowledge is incomplete. We will need to investigate the issue further to reveal other relevant (cultural) knowledge that may extend our understanding of the issue." Expert knowledge, in this case, becomes another resource to be applied to the issue investigated and stands alongside the knowledge and understandings of other people whose deep and extended experience in the setting provides knowledge resources that might usefully be applied to the solution of the problem investigated.

This change in status of the researcher also signals a change in relationships, since the researcher is no longer "boss" or director of the investigation, but acts more like a consultant. In the latter case, research participants may be seen as employers or customers with the right to determine the nature of the research as well as the research processes. As a good business principle, "the customer is always right" signals the nature of the change in relationship between researcher and participants. As John Heron indicates in *Cooperative Inquiry* (1996), "self-directing persons develop most fully through fully reciprocal relations with other self-directing persons. Autonomy and cooperation are necessary and mutually enhancing values of human life. Hence experiential research involves a co-equal relation between two people, reversing the roles of facilitator and agent, or combining them at the same time." As the anthropologist George Marcus (1998) indicated, "[social] affiliations and identities give [research participants] an immense advantage in shaping research . . . There is control of language and a well of life experience that are great assets for achieving the sort of depth [of understanding] that anthropologists have always hoped for from one- to two-year fieldwork projects."

Wadsworth (2001) describes the complex and highly integrated experience required to investigate mental health services at a large central city psychiatric hospital. The study incorporated the perspectives of patients and staff within a consumer organization. The study used multiple sources of information and a reiterative, participatory approach to inquiry that provided deep insight to the experienced reality of people in the hospital. It supplied the means to effect systematic change, including the use of consumers to act as quality improvement consultants in mental health services. She writes of the many micro-skills required to enact this type of work and the major areas of activity required to successfully facilitate collaborative inquiry. The message is clear. Just as carefully controlled and rigorous procedures provide the basis for sound scientific experimentation, so the work of action research requires different, but equally rigorous, activity to translate multiple perspectives and experiences into practical, effective outcomes.

Participatory action research, therefore, enacts systematic inquiry in ways that are:

- Democratic
- Participatory
- Empowering
- Life-enhancing

These changes highlight the nature and exciting potentials of action research, providing opportunities for a worker, clients, colleagues, families, and other stakeholders to engage in exciting and sometimes exhilarating work together. Processes of investigation, therefore, not only provide information and understanding as key outcomes of a process of inquiry, but provide the possibility of enabling people to develop a sense of togetherness, which creates the basis for effective and productive relationships spilling over into all aspects of their life together. As they participate in action research, people develop high degrees of motivation and are often empowered to act in ways they never thought possible. Action research is not only empowering, but provides the basis for building democratic learning communities that enhance the life of agencies, organizations, and institutions.

These characteristics also align action research with the principles of the Alma Ata Declaration on Primary Health Care (PHC), "Health for All" (UNICEF, 1978), and the directives of the Ottawa Charter on Health Promotion (Wass, 2000). By engaging both health service providers and recipients, practitioners establish a foundation for health care that is practical, socially and culturally acceptable, collaborative and accessible, and that encourages self reliance and self-determination—all cardinal principles of PHC. By asserting these principles and answering these imperatives, and thus linking health interventions to the global effort of "Health for All," action research provides practitioners and research participants with a greater purpose that links their practices with others.

Recently, I engaged in an action research process with a neighborhood group in a poorer part of town. Debriefing participants in the latter stages of the process, I was struck by the excitement evident in their lively talk and shining eyes, and the enthusiasm with which they reviewed their experience. "You know, Ernie," said one, "It was such an empowering experience for us." Asked how it had been empowering, she responded, "Because we were able to do it ourselves, instead of having experts come and do it and tell us. We learned so much in the process, and now we know how to do research." She and another woman who participated in the project indicated a desire to extend their understanding of research processes and to extend their skills. Enrolled as extension students, they sat in on my graduate research class, participating actively and providing class participants with great insight into effective ways of practicing action research in community contexts.

This is not an isolated instance as I've shared the excitement and experienced the feelings of accomplishment of young children, teenagers, adminstrators, parents, graduate students, and university professors in large cities, small country towns, and remote communities. My experience encompasses a wide range of social and cultural contexts on two continents, and the power of participatory processes to engage enthusiasm and excitement still excites me. For me, action research is not a dreary, objective, mechanistic process, but a vital, energizing process that engages the mind, enhances the spirit, and creates the unity that enables people to accomplish highly significant goals. At its best, it is a transformational experience enabling people to see the world anew, and in some cases, to literally change their lives.

There is another side to action research, however, that continues to sustain me professionally—the ability to provide the means to accomplish exciting work in the most difficult of circumstances. In a world that has become increasingly alienating by the forces of economic rationalism and accountability, where every activity must be justified in terms of a pre-specified benchmark and justified in dollar terms, the spiritual and artistic side of work life can easily be lost in a maze of technical, mechanistic, and clinical procedure that too easily dulls and nullifies the creative, life-enhancing outcomes of a truly professional experience. The energy and excitement generated by collaborative accomplishment not only provides the means to accomplish the technical, professional goals of our work, but to do so in ways that are truly meaningful and enriching, not only for ourselves, but for the people with whom we work.

Conclusion

Research texts quite often work on an unspoken assumption that applications of the technical routines of scientific research provide the basis for enlightened and improved professional practice. This chapter has suggested the need to broaden ideas about the nature and function of research projects to ensure that they acknowledge and take into account the social and human dimensions of community life. While scientifically validated knowledge truly has the potential to improve our professional practices, it often fails to provide the means to take into account the social, cultural, ethical, and political nature of people's everyday lives.

The participatory and interpretive approach to action research found in this text seeks to provide a more balanced approach to inquiry, providing research procedures that are conducive of democratic and humane social processes within institutions and community contexts. The intent is to provide a rigorous approach to inquiry that legitimizes the perspectives and experiences of all people involved, takes account of scientifically validated information in the processes, and encompasses the means for accomplishing sustainable and effective social and behavioral practices that really make a difference in people's lives.

In the chapters that follow, therefore, the technical routines of research are accomplished within a set of principles that value the human dimensions of professional life. These principles are expressed more clearly in the next chapter, as a precursor to the detailed articulation of action research processes.

SUMMARY

Understanding Action Research:
Exploring Issues of Paradigm and Method

The chapter distinguishes between two major research paradigms: *Objective science*, sometimes called scientific positivism, and *naturalistic inquiry*, often referred to as qualitative or interpretive research.

Objective science assumes a fixed universe that can be observed and explained with precision. Through experimental method, it seeks generalizable information with high degrees of reliability that can be applied across diverse settings. It seeks high degrees of predictability and control.

Naturalistic inquiry focuses on understanding the systems of meaning and interpretation inherent in people's everyday social lives. It makes use of qualitative methods to understand how people experience and make meaning of events.

Action research requires a different set of relationships than those often engaged by professionals. It is a participatory form of inquiry that seeks to make use of the deep-seated and extended understandings people have of their own situations.

Action research embodies a set of social principles that are both democratic and ethical. It seeks to engage processes of inquiry that are democratic, participatory, empowering, and life-enhancing.

Initiating a Study: Research Design

RESEARCH DESIGN	DATA GATHERING	DATA ANALYSIS	COMMUNICATION	ACTION
INITIATING A STUDY	CAPTURING STAKEHOLDER EXPERIENCES AND PERSPECTIVES	IDENTIFYING KEY FEATURES OF EXPERIENCE	WRITING REPORTS	CREATING SOLUTIONS
Setting the stage			Reports	Care plans
			Ethnographies	
Focusing and framing	Interviewing	Analyzing epiphanies and illuminative experiences	Biographies	Case management
	Observing		PRESENTATIONS AND PERFORMANCES	Problem-solving
Literature review				
	Reviewing artifacts	Categorizing and coding	Presentations	Enhancing practices
Stakeholders			Drama	
			Poetry	
Data sources	Reviewing literature	Enhancing analysis	Song	Evaluation
			Dance	
Ethics			Art	Health promotion
		Constructing category frameworks	Video	
Validity			Multimedia	Community development
				Professional development
				Strategic planning

This chapter describes processes for initiating an action research study. Continuing cycles of observation, reflection, and action are presented here as a LOOK, THINK, ACT framework. The chapter discusses the first iteration of the participatory action research cycle—the formulation of the study. The practitioner works with stakeholders to:

- *Create* a productive research environment.
- *Design* the study (i.e., formulate an action plan for the research processes).
- *Focus* the study and state it in researchable terms.
- *Frame* the scope of the inquiry.
- Engage in a preliminary *review of the literature.*
- Identify *sources of data.*
- Describe methods of *data analysis.*
- Take account of *ethical* considerations.
- Establish the *validity* of the study.

Setting the Stage: Creating a Productive Research Environment

As the previous chapter indicates, action research is not just a set of technical procedures providing information to improve curative or care practices. Action research is an *engaged* approach to research that enmeshes health professionals in the lifeworlds of clients, families, and the community. In its best form, action research provides opportunities to develop good working relationships between participants, and, in health terms, the development of a caring community. In such circumstances, health practices become infused with a creative energy that enables people not only to perform to the best of their capabilities, but to engage their full human potential.

As we approach the technical routines of investigation, therefore, it is necessary to articulate the general working principles of action research to maximize the possibility of effective and productive outcomes. The holistic approach to inquiry involves solutions that have the potential to take into account the physical, emotional, aesthetic, spiritual, intellectual, moral, and social life of those involved.

With Head, Heart, and Hand: The Human Dimensions of Action Research

> When we can work with head, heart and hand, we begin to shape a kind of community that is responsive to many different communities, in different places and in different times, and one that opens many ways forward. (Kelly and Sewell, 1988, p. 2.)

Action research can be characterized as "research about practice." Its intent is to enable health professionals to systematically investigate significant problems experienced in their workplaces, with the intent that they identify more effective ways of enacting the work they do with clients and patients. Effective caring practices engage the patient in an active process of diagnosis, providing relevant information, and empowering them to formulate care plans or interventions that not only are effective for the purposes of immediate treatment, but also provide the basis for ongoing sound health behaviors. One of the very productive aspects of both health care and research is the ability to fully engage all dimensions of experience—to employ the heads, hands, and hearts of the people who are involved with the health situation.

The task is not always easy, as practitioners often face clients who are disinterested, fractious, or rebellious, expecting the magic pill that will cure them without any effort or activity on their part. One of the enduring tasks of health practice is to develop and sustain client interest and the expectation that they should actively engage in the processes of attaining and maintaining good health. The intent of an action research process is to generate effective solutions to practical problems by engaging the *heart* or the *spirit* of clients and colleagues, so they do not just go through the motions, but take ownership for their well-being and engage it enthusiastically and creatively. The same is true for health professionals themselves who may use action research to develop and sustain the creative energy required for their demanding day-to-day work with clients.

Professional practitioners sometimes have difficulty imagining that research could make such a difference to their work life. As a university instructor, however, I have discovered the energy emerging from participatory processes of inquiry. Over the past decades, I have been humbled by the sometimes impassioned comments of professional practitioners who have embraced the tenets of action research and applied them to their work situations. Often working in the most difficult of situations, they have been able to transform their professional lives, engaging the creative energies of clients, families, and community people. One practitioner, engaging this form of research for the first time, commented, "It has been a long time since I have had a paradigmatic shift like this in such a profound way. [It] is like a small earthquake or miniature shock of lightning arousing me from my day-to-day automatic pilot semi-slumber." This type of response from people with whom I work in institutional and community settings continues to sustain my excitement and enthusiasm. The technical routines I learn and teach are important, but the processes by which they become instilled in people's experience is a central ingredient of a truly rewarding experience.

One of the problems of engaging the "heart" of clients, however, lies in the complexity practitioners face in their daily work lives. Our work alongside Australian Aboriginal people, whose needs are often quite different from the mainstream population, has sensitized us to this facet of public life. These experiences have been reinforced by work in North American, Asian, and European contexts, where Asian, African American, Hispanic, and indigenous ethnic groups in rural, remote, and inner city contexts provide a rich tapestry of humanity that not only holds a fertile cultural resource, but challenges practitioners to accommodate the diversity that exists in their workplaces. Often, the complexity of these situations encourages us to ignore the implicit differences in our clients, speaking of them in technical or objectifying language—"the patient" or "the client"—and characterizing their failure to accomplish health or treatment outcomes in terms of personal inadequacies like laziness or deviance. We often focus on "interventions" or "strategies" to repair their inappropriate or inadequate performances without acknowledging the possibility of engaging the resourcefulness of the people with whom we work.

The approach to action research presented in this book works on the assumption that people, even very young people, have deep and extended understandings of their lives, enabling them to negotiate their way through an often bewildering and unpredictable life-world. It is our willingness to acknowledge the legitimacy of their world-views, and the wisdom, that enables them to survive and sometimes thrive in difficult circumstances that is at the heart of the participatory processes described in this book. The use of interviews as a central component of action research enables us to listen carefully to what people say, to record and represent events in their own terms, and to use their perceptions and interpretations in formulating plans and activities. The task is not to convince them of the inadequacies of their perspective, but to find ways of enabling them, through sharing each other's perspectives, to formulate more productive under-standings of their own situation.

This orientation to research, therefore, seeks to enhance people's feelings of competence and worth, engaging them in processes that provide an affirmation of themselves, their friends, their families, and their communities. Our work with others—clients, colleagues, families, and administrators—enables them to main-tain a constructive vision of themselves, anchoring them in a productive perspec-tive of their worlds, and enabling them to work easily and comfortably with those around them. Engaging the heart means caring, in an ongoing way, with those facets of human experience that make a difference in the quality of their day-to-day lives. When we talk of the heart of the matter, or engaging the heart of the people, we are talking about their feelings of pride, dignity, identity, responsibil-ity, and locatedness (Figure 3.1).

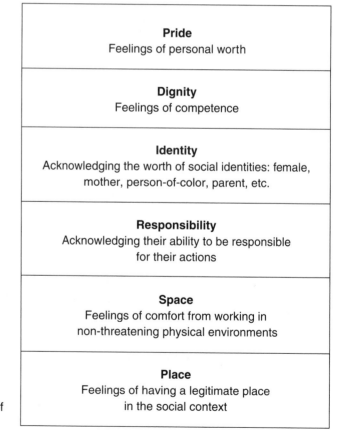

Figure 3.1
The Human Dimensions of
Action Research

The energy and joy emerging from research processes that hear the voices of the people, engage their knowledge and skills, and enable them to actively participate in the construction of activities, events, projects, programs, and services have been an integral part of my professional experience for many years. When I see people talk with shining eyes of their accomplishments, when I see them deeply engaged in work affecting their lives, when I see them moved to upgrade and extend their well-being, and continue to move in often-difficult terrain over extended periods, I know that their hearts have been engaged. They rarely do so in isolation, however; the work they accomplish is enhanced by the common unity they share with those with whom they have worked.

Research Planning and Design

The first step in a research process is to construct a preliminary picture of the project. Practitioners will work with other stakeholders to construct this picture and refine the detail of their research activities. As they commence the work of inquiry, they will design the research and detail an action plan listing the steps to be taken.

- **Building a preliminary picture:** Identifying the research problem and the people affected by or having an affect on the problem.
- **Focusing:** Refining the statement of the research problem, the research question, and research objectives.
- **Framing:** Establishing the scope of the inquiry.
- **Sampling:** Procedures for identifying project participants.
- **Sources of information/data:** Identifying stakeholding groups, sites and settings, statistical records, and other sources of documentary information providing input to the study.
- **Form of the information/data:** The type of information that will inform the inquiry—interview transcripts, observational records, review summaries, televisual documentaries, formal research reports, clinical records, and so on.
- **Data gathering:** How information will be gathered—including interviews, focus groups, observations, reviewing reports and records, reviewing materials and equipment, and so on.
- **Data analysis:** Ways of distilling information to identify key features, concepts, or meanings—for example, event analysis, categorizing, and coding.
- **Ethics:** Steps taken to ensure that no harm is done to people through their inclusion in the research.
- **Validity:** Procedures used to enhance the strength of the research.

Building the Researcher's Picture: The Reflective Practitioner

The initial processes of focusing, framing, and designing an action research study—constituted here as the first of a number of cycles of observation, reflection, and action—may be depicted as a Look-Think-Act sequence that is easily understood by a lay audience.

In the first research cycle, practitioners carefully observe relevant settings (Look), then reflect on their observations to clarify the nature of the research problem (Think). They identify the people who will be involved, and with them develop an initial plan (Act) that incorporates the focus of investigation, the research question, and the scope of the inquiry. Continuing cycles of the Look-Think-Act process enable the practitioner-researcher and other participants to further refine the details of their investigation.

> LOOK entails building a preliminary picture of the situation, enabling the researcher to describe *who* is involved, *what* is happening, and *how, where, and when* events and activities occur. Information is acquired by observing, interacting, and talking informally with people.
>
> THINK requires researchers to reflect on the emerging picture. It is a preliminary analysis of the situation enabling researchers to develop a clearer understanding of what is happening, how it is happening, and the stakeholding groups affected by or affecting the issue.
>
> ACT defines the actions emerging from reflection. It requires people to *plan* their next steps and *implement* appropriate activity. *Evaluation* of these steps requires another cycle of the Look-Think-Act process.

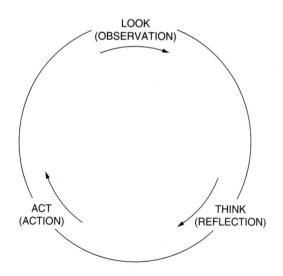

Figure 3.2
The Look-Think-Act
Research Cycle

Focusing the Study

It is not always easy to identify where a study should begin, since problems tend to occur as an interrelated series of issues and events. Specific health problems are often associated with poor diet, inadequate living conditions, lack of exercise, negative attitudes, and so on. Trying to define what is *the* problem can easily become a "chicken-and-egg" process having no particular beginning or end, or no clearly defined cause-and-effect relationships.

Sometimes our first analysis of a situation focuses on related events that prove to be peripheral to the problem about which we are concerned. A recent meeting of a community organization I attended focused on the problem of lack of community participation, with the executive committee discussing ways of increasing the involvement level of local people. Eventually, I asked committee members whether, in fact, participation was the real problem, and asked them to consider the problem behind the problem. They spoke of a number of issues about which they were concerned, including the failure of people to engage in required actions to remediate the conditions or situations from which they were suffering. In this case, the problem upon which the community initially focused—participation—turned out to be multidimensional, participation being one facet of more deep-seated problems. Once the underlying problems were identified, the board was able to reflect more broadly on the issues about which they were concerned. The problem of participation, in fact, turned out to be a suggested solution to the underlying problems. In the first stages of research, therefore, research participants need to carefully reflect on the nature of "the problem" about which they are concerned.

One of the major strengths of action research is its emergent quality—its ability to allow researchers to tentatively state the problem, then refine and reframe the study by continuing iterations of the Look-Think-Act research cycle. In a study instigated by the managers of a local health service, for instance, the researcher was told that alcohol was a major problem for the community. The researcher facilitated a discussion among the managers and some employees guided by the question, "What do we want to know about alcohol?" A specific question emerged from the group discussion, "What effects does alcohol have in our community?" The group decided that an investigation of the experience of alcohol in a sample of households was necessary. The young health workers who were to conduct the investigation needed to find a way to enter households in a respectful way to investigate this question. After a series of role plays in which they rehearsed the scenario of entering the households, the health workers framed their research question within the rationale of their professional healing role. The research question became, "What suffering is experienced in your household as a result of alcohol?"

The initial stages of focusing the research and formulating a researchable question are essentially reflective processes, requiring practitioners to engage in conversations with other stakeholders and to think carefully through all dimensions of the issue causing concern. The first step is to reflect carefully on what is happening that is problematic and what issues and events are related to that problem. To focus the research more clearly, the issue or problem is stated in the form of a researchable question, and the objective of studying that issue is identified. These should be clearly stated as follows[1]:

- The *issue or topic* to be studied: Defining which issues or events are causing concern.
- The *research problem*: Stating the issue as a problem.
- The *research question*: Reframing that problem as a question—asking, in effect, "What is happening here?"
- The *research objective*: Describing what we would hope to achieve by studying this question.[2]

Sheila Jones's study of patient care was defined in the following terms:

Issue: Patients are consistently failing to comply with their care plan, resulting in failure to progress.
Problem: The patients are failing to carry our their care plans.
Question: How do patients experience and understand their care plans?
Objective: To understand how patients experience and understand their care plans.

The preliminary reflective process for developing the focus of the study is assisted by dialogue with both potential participants and colleagues. While it is possible that the research focus may later change as other participants pose their own particular questions, the initiator of the project should be clear about the significance of their own research questions. The initial development of the research question should focus on **how** participants and other stakeholders experience the

---

[1] Since this is a qualitative research study, a research hypothesis—a suggested answer to the research question—is not part of the design. Qualitative or interpretive inquiry is hypothesis generating, rather than hypothesis testing. "Testing" of the "hypotheses" generated by an action research process is accomplished through continual cycling through the Look-Think-Act routine, so that actions put into place as a result of the first cycle of investigation are subject to evaluative processes through further observation and analysis—Looking and Thinking.

[2] Qualitative studies usually focus on *understanding* people's experience and perspectives as a common outcome of the research process. Quantitative or experimental studies, on the other hand, more often focus on *explanations* that explain how one group of variables is associated with other variables.

problematic issue and **how** they interpret events and other information. How is it that these health problems occur? How do clients perceive that they manage their care plans? In action research, the focus is largely on events and their interpretation rather than factual information of strongly developed causal connections explaining "why" events occur.

By developing a clear, precise, and focused research question, research participants take an essential reference point into their inquiry. As investigations proceed, they are able to evaluate the emerging data according to its reference to the research question(s). The initial research question should be shared by all participants and reiterated consistently throughout the research cycles as a constant guide to investigation.

Framing the Study: Delimiting the Scope of the Inquiry

Before commencing, research participants will make decisions about the sample of people to be included in the study, the sites or settings in which the research will take place, and the times the research activities will take place. Decisions will also be made about the extent of participation by those involved in the study, defining who will be involved in the various research activities and who will monitor and support people in their research work.

These considerations run hand-in-hand with the need to consider the breadth of issues to be incorporated into the study as they emerge. Too many issues may make the study complex and unwieldy, but restricting the study may cause issues to be neglected that have an important bearing on the problem. In the Koch and Kralich (2002) study, for instance (see Chapter 1), the group of women living with multiple sclerosis initially explored a broad range of issues. As the study developed, however, they focused more particularly on ways of improving their management of incontinence. In this instance, they were able to identify specific strategies for managing incontinence and improving the quality of their lives.

Researchers, therefore, will initially broadly identify:

- **What:** What is the problem requiring investigation? What is my central research question?
- **Who:** Who are the likely stakeholders? Which people are affected by or have an affect on the issue being studied? Nurses? Physicians? Administrators? Family members? Others?
- **Place:** Where will the research take place? Which sites or settings will be included in the study? Clinics? Hospitals? Offices? Homes? Other locations?
- **Time:** When will the research begin? How long might it take?
- **Scope:** What is the likely scope of the investigation? Client treatment? Client short-term care? Long-term care? Prevention? and so on.

Once practitioners have assisted research participants in clarifying the focus, frame, and scope of the research, they will undertake a preliminary search to identify other perspectives on the issue embedded in the literature. This may assist them to further clarify the nature and extent of their investigations.

Preliminary Literature Review

As Creswell (2002) points out, literature reviews for qualitative research have different purposes than those in quantitative research. While substantial use of the literature provides the basis for formulating a quantitative study, qualitative studies use the literature review quite minimally in the earlier phases of a study. Since the latter focuses on stakeholder experiences and perspectives, pre-formulation of the issue according to concepts and analyses in the literature is deemed inappropriate. Because of the nature of qualitative research, initial conceptions of the research are always assumed to be provisional, thus limiting the possibility of an exhaustive review of the literature. The preliminary literature review, therefore, serves three main purposes: It alerts research participants to others who have studied similar issues, it may assist to refine the research question, and it may provide insights into methods of investigation.

Understandings and information emerging from the literature, however, may augment, complement, or challenge stakeholder perspectives as the study progresses. Since health issues have been the subject of study for many decades, research participants may increase the power of their investigation by reviewing literature that speaks to emerging concepts and issues. In some cases, they may identify potential solutions to the problems that have been successfully enacted in other contexts, or acquire information that clarifies issues emerging in the study. Frequently, salient issues emerging in the data collection phase influence the direction of the investigation, causing participants to pursue different but related questions. Hence, the literature search will evolve as an ongoing feature of the research process, emerging in accordance with the directions and agendas indicated by participant-constructed descriptions of the situation.

Literature Search

The first phase of a search requires researchers to identify relevant literature. This task is greatly enhanced by the capabilities of computer-assisted search engines available in most libraries. It will be necessary to identify three to four key concepts related to the issue to feed into the search routine. Where large numbers of items are identified, it may be necessary to delineate further key concepts to narrow the search to the most relevant sources of information. Perusing annotated collections that provide a brief description of the content of the reading may enhance this process.

An increasing body of material is available on the web that provides researchers with useful resources for their study. Sole reliance on the web, however, is not recommended, as the information available from this source tends to be incomplete and patchy. As in library searches, researchers will need to identify key concepts to feed into the search process.

Researchers often distinguish between:

- **Primary sources** providing direct reports of original research
- **Secondary sources** that report on or summarize primary source material
- **Professional literature** based on the perspectives of experienced professionals
- **Institutional reports** from government or institutional authorities
- **Practice literatue** presenting or advocating particular approaches to professional practice

University and professional libraries provide a wide variety of relevant literature, including theses and dissertations, journals, books, handbooks, abstracts, and encyclopedias. Library staff can often assist in identifying initial reading pertinent to the problem being investigated, but review of any material will identify other sources of information so that a review of the literature becomes an ever-expanding search. Researchers should note sources cited in journal articles, research reports, and texts, then review those for further information.

Identifying Different Perspectives in the Literature

The preliminary literature review extends the think/reflect part of the research cycle, providing new possibilities for conceptualizing or interpreting the issue. The preliminary search, therefore, should be sufficiently broad to provide researchers with an understanding of the different perspectives and types of information presented within the literature. These will not only differ according to the disciplines of the authors—psychology, sociology, cultural studies, and so on—but according to different theoretical positions from within each discipline. The literature may also vary according to the formal and informal reports from a variety of institutional sources, including clinic, district, state, and national documents. It may include video/television documentaries, as well as information on projects and activities available on the web.

As the project progresses, participants will select, review, and evaluate relevant literature as part of the processes of data collection, identifying pertinent information to enhance the understandings emerging from other sources (see Chapter 4, page 84). Studies by other people within the literature become other perspectives (or stakeholders) to be incorporated into the process of data collection and analysis. The preliminary review of the literature within the first iteration of the action research cycle is conducted through the lens of the initial research question, alerting participants to other studies about similar problems, assisting with the refinement of the research question, and/or providing insight into research methods.

Sampling: Selecting Participants

The purpose of sampling is to ensure that the particular assumptions and understandings of people involved in a specific context are taken into account in seeking effective solutions to the issue studied. In most studies, limits on time and resources make it impossible to include *all* people who might potentially inform the research process, so it is necessary to select a smaller group to provide the information (data) on which the research is grounded. A technique called *purposive,* or *purposeful, sampling* seeks to ensure that the diverse perspectives of people likely to affect the issue are included in the study. Creswell (2002) suggests that purposive sampling seeks to select participants for a variety of purposes. These include:

- People who represent the diverse perspectives found in any social context (maximal variation sampling)
- Particularly troublesome or enlightening cases (extreme case sampling)

- Participants who are "typical" of people in the setting (typical sampling)
- Participants who have particular knowledge related to the issue studied (theory or concept sampling)

In all cases, researchers need to purposively select a sample of participants that represents the variation of perspectives and experiences across all groups and sub-groups who affect or are affected by the issue under investigation—the stakeholders in the study.[3]

The first task is to identify the primary stakeholding groups[4]—that is the group most centrally involved or affected by the issue studied. If a study is concerned about youth engaging in risky health behaviors, the youth themselves would be a primary stakeholding group, while a study of patient participation in the development of care plans would have patients as a primary stakeholders. Sometimes the primary stakeholding groups are complementary groups. A study of a care issue might include nurses and patients as primary stakeholders, while a study of patient care plans might include care-givers, clients and family.

> An action research inquiry into the activities of a community health service identified community health nurses as the primary reference group. Clients, physicians, clinical nurses, transport drivers, and welfare workers were also included as stakeholders.

The next task is to identify, within those stakeholding groups, the different types or groups of people likely to have an affect on or be affected by the issue studied. Issues of gender, class, race, and ethnicity are paramount, since these factors are likely to be related to significant variation in experience and perspective. Researchers might need to ensure that men and women are included in their sample, that poorer clients are represented as well as those from more middle-class backgrounds, and that each racial and ethnic group in the client group is included. Depending on the context, it may be necessary for researchers to include members of different social cliques, religious affiliations, sporting groups, or other types of groups represented in the social setting.

---

[3] Purposive sampling differs in nature and purpose from random sampling used for experimental studies. A random sample drawn from a larger population enables experimental researchers to use statistical procedures to generalize from that sample to a larger population. Rather than seeking to generalize, action research seeks solutions to problems and questions that are quite context specific.

[4] In some literature the *primary stakeholding group* is referred to as the *critical reference group*. The intent, however, is similar—to focus on those primarily affected by the issue studied.

> An older woman attended an action research project discussion group focusing on drug abuse in a rural community. While more articulate middle-aged people readily articulated their viewpoints on the nature and scope of the problem, she remained very quiet. However, in a quiet moment, she spoke of her own anguish and suffering when caring for grandchildren who seemed to have lost respect for their elders. Her story added a previously unrecognized dimension to the issue.

While it is not always possible to include people from *all* groups in any setting, those selected should include participants from groups likely to have a significant impact on the issue studied, or those on whom the issue is likely to have the most impact. To fail to include participants because it is not convenient, because they show little interest, or because they are non-communicative is to put the effectiveness of the study at risk. The previous chapter talked of the need to establish research relationships to maximize the possibility of including everyone likely to affect the issue studied.

It is not always possible for researchers to nominate in advance those who need to be included in a study. A technique called *snowballing* enables researchers to ask participants who they think needs to be included, or to ask someone they might nominate who has quite a different perspective or set of experiences related to the issue studied. In this way, researchers commence by defining likely participants, but extend their sample to be more inclusive of the diverse and significant perspectives included in the study.

Any group, however, is likely to include people who are natural leaders, or who in some way are able to sway the opinions or perspectives of others in their group—sometimes referred to as opinion leaders. Researchers should try to ensure that the sample selected includes both natural leaders and opinion leaders. A general rule of thumb in this process is to ask "Who can speak for this group? Whose word will group members acknowledge as representing their perspective?" The research design may not specify a particular sample, but will describe the procedures for identifying those who will be active participants in the study.

Later stages of a study related to the development of a new program or service may use standard survey techniques to check the validity of information gained in the first phases of the study, or to gain new information related to potential users of those programs and services. In these instances, standard procedures for selecting a random sample from the population of interest will apply (see Chapter 4).

Sources and Forms of Information (Data Gathering)

Participants need to define the types of information enabling them to work toward a resolution of the issue or to accomplish the tasks of an action research process. Participant perspectives, experiences, and events will constitute a significant portion of the data, captured in the form of accounts providing descriptions of the qualities of the problem or the issue being investigated. The major source of information in action research usually is that provided by interviewing stakeholding research participants—the sample described previously.

Other sources of information, however, complement participant accounts, including information from records, scientifically grounded studies, or the stock of knowledge provided by the health sciences—anatomy, physiology, medication, and so on. Some of this will be incorporated into the study through the inputs provided by health professionals, but research participants may also observe or review a variety of other sources to acquire relevant information. Common sources of information include cultural settings (places), events, activities, materials and equipment, work samples, documents, records, reports, relevant literature, and so on (see Chapter 4, page 79). Data is collected from these sources by observation of settings and events or by reviewing documentary and other recorded information.

The research design, therefore, should stipulate the type of data to be acquired and the methods employed to access different types of information, including interviews, focus groups, observations, reviews, photographs, video-recording, and audio-recording. Structured interviews, questionnaires, and observation schedules may also be used in the later stages of a project. Because of the emergent nature of qualitative research, it is not possible to signal precisely all sources of information in advance, but the design should provide participants with guidance about where, when, how, and from whom initial information will be acquired.

Distilling Information (Analyzing the Data)

A research design informs participants and those reading research proposals of the data analysis methods used in the study. The research design should clearly signal the type of data analysis employed and the use to which analyzed data might be applied to actions emerging in the latter stages of the study (see Chapter 5, pages 91 and 103).

RESEARCH DESIGN

Being an essentially qualitative approach to inquiry, an action research design provides the following information:

1. *Focus:* A statement of the issue, the research problem, the research question, and research objective(s).
2. *Framing the scope of inquiry:* The place, the time, the stakeholding groups, and the scope of the issues included in the study.
3. *Preliminary literature review:* Processes for reviewing the literature.
4. *Sources of information/data:* The stakeholders, sites and settings, and literature from which information will be acquired.
5. *Data gathering processes:* Ways information will be gathered—interviews, observation, review of materials and equipment, and so on.
6. *Data analysis processes:* Procedures used for distilling information.

Research Ethics

The research design also includes ethical protocols that protect the well-being and interests of research participants. Punch (1994) suggests that "the view that science is intrinsically neutral and essentially beneficial disappeared with the revelations at the Nuremberg trials." Some well-known studies have shown that researchers are not always aware of potential harm that may come to those who participate in research studies (e.g., Horowitz, 1970; Milgram, 1963). Universities, agencies, and organizations usually have explicit guidelines about the ethical conduct of research. In these circumstances, formal research studies must gain explicit approval from an institutional review board, or similar body, prior to conducting their research. The research design needs to specifically address situations of potential harm and include procedures ensuring the safety of participants. As Sieber (1992) indicates, sound ethics and sound methodology go hand in hand.

Confidentiality, Care, and Sensitivity

When people talk for extended periods, they often speak of very private matters, reveal highly problematic events, or even potentially harmful information. A prime directive of social research is to protect the anonymity of participants. In practice, it is best to assume that *all* information acquired is highly confidential. Where we require information to be shared with other participants or audiences, we must first ask relevant participants for permission to do so. When I read back my field notes, or share analyzed information with participants, I ask, "Is there anything here you would not like to reveal to other people in this project?" If they appear unsure, I inform them that it may be possible to present the information but to disguise its source. We can do this by using fictitious names or by reporting it generally—"Some people suggest that. . . . " "Other participants provide a different perspective. . . . "

Aligned with confidentiality is the duty of care we have to participants. We need to ensure that information is stored securely so that others do not inadvertently see it. We certainly should not share recorded information with others without permission of the persons concerned, even if that information points to apparently harmful events in the person's life—drug abuse, physical abuse, and so on. This points to another possibility occasionally arising in the processes of extended interview, where the recall of distressing events creates a deep emotional response. Duty of care requires researchers to provide sufficient time for the person to "debrief" by talking through issues or events to a point of comfort, or by putting them in contact with a family member or counselor who can assist them to resolve the situation.

Permissions

An issue that is currently debated as a result of current moves to engage clients in action research processes as part of their care processes is whether or not formal permission from authorities is required. Though it has yet to be tested legally, some opinions suggest that formal permission is not required when a health professional assists a client to engage in processes of inquiry as part of their ongoing care or treatment. In that case, normal duty-of-care requirements would apply, the professional ensuring that procedures would not put the client at risk. Where they engage in more extended studies that go outside the direct professional-client relationship, possibly involving other health professionals, other clients, or families, formal permissions would need to be obtained prior to commencement of the project. To the extent that the research becomes a public process where people's privacy or personal well-being is at risk, enactment of standard research ethics protocols with a relevant authority is warranted.

Where research is associated with a university course or program, the institution itself will usually have processes for reviewing research through an ethics committee or institutional review board. A similar system operates in clinics, hospitals, and agencies. Though the procedures are sometimes unwieldy and time consuming, they provide a means of ensuring that people's privacy is not violated, and that research processes do not threaten the participants' well-being.

Institutional Ethical Protocols

Research ethics procedures differ between institutions and agencies, but common protocols contain:

- A signed and dated application form
- A description of the proposed research, clearly identified and dated, together with relevant with supporting documents
- A page description of the ethical considerations involved in the research
- Questionnaires or other research materials intended for research participants
- Investigators curriculum vitae, dated and signed
- A description of the process used to obtain and document participants' consent
- Written forms or other research information provided to potential participants
- An informed consent form clearly identified and dated
- A statement describing any compensation to be given to research participants
- A description of the arrangements for insurance coverage for research participants, if applicable
- A statement of agreement to comply with ethical principles set out in relevant guidelines

Informed Consent

In many contexts, protocols require those facilitating research to engage processes of informed consent. This requires the research facilitator and others engaged in data gathering to:

- Inform each participant of the purpose and nature of the study
- Ask whether they wish to participate
- Ask permission to record information they provide
- Assure them of the confidentiality of that information

- Advise them that they may withdraw at any stage and have their recorded information returned
- Ask them to sign a short document affirming their permission

The following document provides an example of how these processes are presented to participants and documented. A consent form not only provides information but is also a record of consent so copies should be provided to each signatory.

AGREEMENT TO PARTICIPATE

Research Study: Services Provided by Community Health Nurses

Researcher: Jeanette Williams   **Phone:** 335-1713

Background

Community health nurses have been employed since the early 1970s to assist in the care of people in their own homes or community settings. They have many demands placed upon them and work in many different situations. They provide many services as part of a community health team, working alongside physicians, clinical nurses, and other health professionals. Although it is important that everyone knows the role of each worker in a team, some confusion has arisen in Burtville about the different responsibilities of community health nurses and other health professionals.

This research seeks to discover:

1. What are the principal tasks of all community health nurses?
2. What are the specialist tasks in which only some community health nurses engage?

Knowing about these things will give information about:

1. The skills in which all community health nurses need training.
2. Specialist training needed by some community health nurses.

The information in this project will largely be collected by observing community health nurses and talking with them about their work. Researchers will also talk with the nurses' clients. As the information is collected from each person or group of people, reports will be written and shared with the respondents, all names and place names being changed to avoid identification of individuals. Participants will be required to engage in two interviews of about one hour's duration. The researcher also will have a follow-up session with each person to check the accuracy of the information.

Names will be kept confidential. Tape recordings and field notes always will be stored in a secure place by the researcher and not used for purposes other than the current study. Photographs will only be used with written permission.

If you wish to withdraw from the study at any time, you are free to do so and, if you wish, all information you have given will be shredded or returned. If you wish to contact the research coordinator at any time, you may contact her at the above phone number.

I _____ have read the information above and any questions I have asked have been answered to my satisfaction. I agree to participate in this activity on the understanding that I may withdraw at any time without prejudice. I agree that the research data generated may be published provided my name is not used or that I am not otherwise identified.

Signed _____ (participant) _____ Date
Signed _____ (facilitator) _____ Date

RESEARCH ETHICS

Ethical procedures are established by:

1. *Confidentiality:* Privacy is protected by ensuring confidentiality of information.
2. *Permissions:* Permission is obtained to carry out the research from appropriate authorities.
3. *Informed consent:* Participants are informed of the nature of the study and provide formal consent to be included.

Validity in Action Research: A Question of Quality

When health practitioners engage in research directly related to their work, they are usually able to ascertain the worth of research according to its usefulness in helping them accomplish their professional tasks. Studies wider in scope, however, involving official approval or requests for funding often need to satisfy more stringent requirements. People want assurance that sloppy, poorly devised, or unbalanced research is not likely to result in inadequate or potentially damaging outcomes. In these circumstances, they often require an examination of the rigor or strength of the procedures to be included in the research design sections of a proposal; or in the methodology section of a research report.

Action research, being essentially qualitative or naturalistic, seeks to construct holistic understandings of the dynamic and complex social world of clinic or agency. It reveals people's subjective experiences and the ways they meaningfully construct and interpret events, activities, behaviors, responses, and problems. Although these types of studies provide powerful understandings enabling the development of effective practices and activities, they are mostly specific to particular contexts and lack stability over time—what is true at one time may vary as policies and procedures shift and the actors in the setting change. When a new administrator is appointed to a clinic, or staff changes occur, for instance, then professional life in that context is likely to change in significant ways. The same is true when changes occur in organizational objectives, policies, and procedures. Because of the constant flux in conditions and personnel, the truths emerging from naturalistic inquiry are always contingent (i.e., they are "true" only for the people, the time and setting of that particular study). We are not looking for "the Truth" or "the causes," but "truths-in-context."

Procedures for evaluating the rigor of experimental or survey research evolve around well-formulated processes for testing reliability[5] and establishing the validity[6] of a study. Traditional experimental criteria for establishing validity, however, are inappropriate for qualitative action research, and debate continues about a broadly acceptable set of criteria to use for this purpose. Some researchers have approached this task by seeking to identify the foundational assumptions underlying the term validity. "What does it mean?" they ask, "When we seek to establish the 'validity' of a study?" Two highly respected scholars, Denzin and Lincoln (1998b, p. 414), interpret validity as follows:

> . . . a text's call to authority and truth . . . is established through recourse to a set of rules concerning knowledge, its production, and representation. The rules, as Scheurich (1992, p. 1) notes, if properly followed, establish validity. Without validity there is not truth, and without truth there can be not trust in a text's claims to validity. . . . validity becomes a boundary line that 'divides good research from bad, separates acceptable (to a particular research community) research from unacceptable research. . . .' (Scheurich, 1992, p. 5).

Trustworthiness

Because qualitative methods are essentially subjective in nature and local in scope, procedures for assessing the validity of research are quite different than those used for experimental study. As the previous quote suggests, a new set of criteria are required to provide people with trust that the research is acceptable. Lincoln and Guba

---

[5] Reliability is estimated by measures of the extent to which similar results may be expected from similar samples within the population studied, across different contexts, and at different times. Reliability focuses on the stability of results across time, settings, and samples.

[6] Experimental validity is defined in two ways—external validity and internal validity. Measures of external validity estimate the probability that results obtained from the sample differ significantly from results we would expect. Internal validity focuses on the extent to which results obtained might be attributed to the dependant variables included in the study and not some other cause. Researchers ask, "Do our instruments actually measure what we wish them to measure?" and "Are the results attributal to the dependant variables we have stipulated, or to some other related variable?" Internal validity focuses on careful research, design, and instrumentation. Both reliability and validity are verified by statistical and other techniques.

(1985) provide a common set of criteria for establishing the validity of qualitative research. They suggest that because there can be no objective measures of validity, the underlying issue is to identify ways of establishing *trustworthiness*, the extent to which we can trust the truthfulness or adequacy of a research project. They propose that establishing trustworthiness involves procedures for attaining:

- **Credibility:** The plausibility and integrity of a study
- **Transferability:** Whether results might be applied to other contexts than the research setting
- **Dependability:** Where research processes are clearly defined and open to scrutiny
- **Confirmability:** Where the outcomes of the study are demonstrably drawn from the data

Trustworthiness, therefore, is established by recording and reviewing the research procedures themselves to establish the extent to which they ensure the phenomena studied is accurately and adequately represented. The following procedures are adapted from those suggested by Lincoln and Guba (1985).

Credibility

Qualitative research is easily open to sloppy, biased processes that merely reinscribe the biases and perspectives of those in control of the research process. Careful adherence to the following processes assists researchers in minimizing the extent to which their own viewpoints intrude. They may also review and record the following features of the research process to provide evidence of rigorous procedure and to enhance the plausibility of their findings.

Prolonged engagement   Brief visits to a research site provide only superficial understandings of events. A rigorous study requires researchers to invest sufficient time to achieve a relatively sophisticated understanding of a context: to learn the intricacies of cultural knowledge and meaning that sustain people's actions and activities in a setting. Prolonged engagement in a setting also enables researchers to establish relationships of trust with participants, which allows them to gain greater access to the "insider" knowledge rather than the often superficial or purposeful information given to strangers. Researchers, therefore, add to the credibility of a study by recording the time spent in the research context.

Persistent observation   Being present in the research context for an extended time period is not a sufficient condition to establish credibility, however. Sometimes researchers mistake their presence in the field for engagement in research. In a recent study, one investigator indicated he had worked with a group of teachers for months. However, he had not engaged in systematic research at that time, and his "observations" were undirected, unfocused, and unrecorded. Participants need to consciously engage in data collection activities to provide depth to their inquiries. This is essential to interviewing processes, as a single interview lasting 15–20 minutes provides very superficial understandings that lack both detail and adequacy. Prolonged engagement signals the need for repeated, extended interviews to establish the adequacy, accuracy, and appropriateness of research materials. Researchers, therefore, need to record the number and duration of observations and interviews.

Triangulation Triangulation involves the use of multiple and different sources, methods, and perspectives to corroborate, elaborate, or illuminate the research problem and its outcomes. It enables the inquirer to clarify meaning by identifying different ways the phenomenon is being perceived (Stake, 1994). In action research, we include all stakeholders relevant to the issue investigated, observe multiple sites and events relevant to the stakeholders and issue investigated, and review all relevant materials, including resources, reports, records, research literature, and so on. These multiple sources and methods provide a rich resource for building adequate and appropriate accounts and understandings that form the base for working toward the resolution of research problems.

Participant debriefing This process is similar to *peer debriefing* as proposed by Lincoln and Guba (1985), but differs because of the researcher's change in status in an action research process. It is not solely the research facilitator who is in need of debriefing, but other participants in the process as well. Debriefing is a process of exposing oneself to a disinterested person for the purpose of exploring and challenging aspects of the inquiry that might otherwise remain only implicit within the participant's mind (Lincoln & Guba, 1985). The purposes of debriefing are to review the appropriateness of research procedures and to clarify the participant ways of describing and interpreting events. Debriefing also provides participants with an opportunity for catharsis, enabling them to deal with emotions and feelings that might cloud their vision or prevent relevant information from emerging. Researcher-facilitators often provide debriefing sessions with research participants, but may also require an interested colleague to engage in debriefing them on the processes of research they are guiding. The credibility of a study is enhanced where researchers record opportunities given to participants to debrief.

Diverse case analysis In all research, it is necessary to ensure that other interpretations of the data are fully explored. Sometimes there is a temptation to include in a research process only those people who are positively inclined toward the issue under study, or to interpret the information in particular ways. Diverse case analysis seeks to ensure that all possible perspectives are taken into account, and that interpretations of important, significant, or powerful people do not overwhelm others. Diverse case analysis enables participants to constantly refine interpretations so that all participant perspectives are included in the final report, and all issues are dealt with. The credibility of a study is enhanced if researchers can demonstrate that all perspectives affecting the study have been included. A clear statement of sampling procedures assists in this process.

Referential adequacy Referential adequacy refers to the need for concepts and structures of meaning within the study to clearly reflect the perspectives, perceptions, and language of participants. When participants' experiences and perspectives are reinterpreted through the lenses of other existing reports or theories, or in terms derived from existing practices, procedures, or policies, research outcomes are likely to be distorted. One of the key features of qualitative research is the need to ensure that interpretations are experience-near, and grounded in the language and terminology used by participants to frame and describe their experience. Where it is necessary to use more general terms to refer to a number of phenomena, those terms should adequately describe the specific details to which they refer. The credibility of a study is enhanced to the extent researchers can demonstrate that outcomes of the study have a direct relationship to the terminology and language used by participants.

Member checks In experimental inquiry, research subjects rarely have the opportunity to question or review the information gathered and the outcomes of the study. The practical nature of action research, however, requires that participants be given frequent opportunity to review the raw data, the analyzed data, and reports that are produced. This process of review is called *member checking* and provides the means for ensuring that the research adequately and accurately represents the perspectives and experiences of participants. Member checking is one of the key procedures required to establish the credibility of a study.

Transferability

Unlike quantitative research that assumes the need to generalize the results of the study, qualitative research by its very nature can only apply results directly to the context of the study. Nevertheless, researchers seek to provide the possibility that results might be transferred to other settings to enable people to take advantage of the knowledge acquired in the course of the study. Whether such application is possible, it is assumed, can be assessed according to the likelihood that another context is sufficiently similar to allow results to be applicable. A study from rural Australia, for instance, may or may not have import for suburban Holland. Qualitative research reports seek to provide sufficiently detailed reports of the context and the participants to enable others to assess the likely applicability of the research to their own situation. Thickly detailed descriptions, therefore, contribute to the trustworthiness of a study by enabling other audiences to clearly understand the nature of the context and the people participating in the study.

Dependability

Trustworthiness also depends on the extent to which observers are able to ascertain whether research procedures are adequate for the purposes of the study. Where insufficient information is available, or available information indicates the likelihood of superficial and/or limited inquiry, they will not feel the study is dependable. The dependability of research is achieved through an *inquiry audit* whereby details of the research process—including processes for defining the research problem, collecting and analyzing data, and constructing reports—are made available to participants and other audiences.

Confirmability

Confirmability is achieved through an audit trail, the inquirer having retained recorded information that can be made available for review. These include raw data such as field notes, photographs, diary entries, original and annotated documents, copies of letters, and materials generated at meetings. They also include data reduction, analysis products, and plans and reports derived from the study. They enable participants or other observers to confirm that research accurately and adequately represents the perspectives presented in the study. This means they enhance the trustworthiness of the study.

Participatory Validity

The credibility of an action research project may also be enhanced by the participation of stakeholders. This overcomes, to some degree, the propensity for researchers to observe and interpret events through the lens of their own interpretive frameworks. A much greater degree of credibility is attained when research participants can check the veracity of the material. As they read the data of their interviews, they are able to verify the accuracy of events described, and as they engage in data analysis, they are able to verify the significant experiences, features, and elements identified. By participating in the construction of reports, they help formulate accounts that more clearly represent their experience and perspective.

Participatory processes respond to recent developments in qualitative research (Altheide & Johnson, 1998) that point to the multiple means now used to establish validity, according to the nature and purposes of the study, and the theoretical frames of reference upon which the research rests. In a very direct way, engaging people as direct participants in the research also enables a study to take into account such issues as emotionality, caring, subjective understanding, and relationships in research (Oleson, 1993, 1998; Lather, 1993) that are important features of feminist research. They are incorporated as a means of ensuring the validity/trustworthiness of a study, but also to enhance the possibility of effective change.

Pragmatic Validity

One of the greatest sources of validity in action research is the utility of the outcomes of research. When participants are able to take effective action on the issue they have investigated, they demonstrate the validity of the research. High degrees of credibility are evident as the understandings that emerge from the processes of inquiry are successfully applied to practical actions. In these circumstances, it becomes evident that emerging concepts and constructions are adequate to account for the phenomena investigated.

ESTABLISHING VALIDITY

The validity of action research is established according to the degree to which an audience can accept it as *trustworthy*. Trustworthiness is established through procedures establishing *credibility, transferability, dependability, confirmability*, degrees of participation, and utility. These are attained through:

1. *Prolonged engagement:* The duration of the research processes.
2. *Persistent observation:* The number and duration of observations and interviews.

3. *Triangulation:* Integration of all sources of data, including the settings observed, the stakeholders interviewed, and materials reviewed.
4. *Participant debriefing:* Processes for reviewing research procedures.
5. *Negative case analysis:* Processes for ensuring a diversity of interpretations is explored.
6. *Referential adequacy:* How terminology within the study is drawn from participant language and concepts.
7. *Member checks:* Procedures for checking the accuracy of data and the appropriateness of data analysis and reporting.
8. *Transferability:* The inclusion of detailed descriptions of the participants and the research context.
9. *Dependability:* Detailed description of the research process.
10. *Confirmability:* The data available for review.
11. *Participation:* The extent of stakeholder participation in the research process.
12. *Utility:* Practical outcomes of the research process.

An Index of Engagement: Excitement, Interest, Apathy, and Resistance

The best action research projects are characterized by high degrees of engagement. Participants talk animatedly, meet frequently to share ideas or explore issues, spend long hours working on activities, work happily, and resolve problems easily and cooperatively. At this level of engagement, **excitement** is evident and highly productive and enjoyable work is a continuing and easily sustainable feature of the situation.

Over time, many projects lose that air of excitement, but participants are able to maintain high degrees of **interest** and to sustain the effectiveness of their work. People work purposively and productively, their talk is easy and collegial as they share ideas and resources, and work collaboratively. Interested participants produce good work that accomplishes the point of the project and gives them high degrees of satisfaction.

Apathy is a common response when people do not see the point of a process, when its purpose is merely ritualistic, or when participants can't see the relevance of research activities. Lethargic interactions are matched by tokenistic responses requiring minimum effort and producing minimum outcomes.

Resistance is a response of people engaged in activities they see as pointless, threatening, or coercive. Goffman (1961) suggests these are common responses in contexts where people have no freedom of choice, or where they are forced to comply with rules over which they have no control. Critical theorists (e.g., Kincheloe & McClaren, 1994) suggest that resistance is a natural response to coercive systems of authority, and that people employ a variety of strategies to alleviate what they consider to be oppressive conditions. Productive work is rarely possible in these situations, and efforts to engage people in any sort of activity focus mainly on systems of reward and punishment to attain required behaviors.

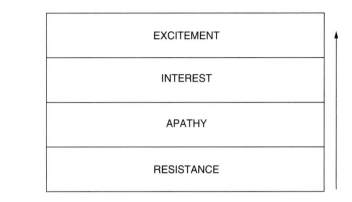

Figure 3.3
Index of Engagement

An Index of Engagement (Figure 3.3) provides a rule-of-thumb measure of the extent to which people are dedicated or committed to the work in hand. By enacting the following principles of action research, researcher-facilitators provide the conditions that maximize the likelihood of interested or excited participants.

Working Principles of Action Research

Four working principles provide the means by which an action research process enables participants to work through the human complexities of a multidimensional process of investigation—relationships, communication, inclusion, and participation. As we engage the technical aspects of research, we need to work in ways that heighten the degree of engagement of participants.

Relationships

Good working relationships enable individuals and groups to trust each other, provide high levels of motivation, and provide the basis for continuing research activities over the sometimes long periods required to deal with significant issues. Good working relationships:

- Promote feelings of equality for all people involved
- Maintain harmony
- Avoid conflicts, where possible
- Resolve conflicts that arise, openly and dialogically
- Accept people as they are, not as some people think they ought to be
- Encourage personal, cooperative relationships, rather than impersonal, competitive, conflictual, or authoritarian relationships
- Are sensitive to people's feelings

Communication

The quality, consistency, and correctness of communication have a vital effect on interactions between individuals and groups. Their work together is likely to be short-lived or ineffectual if people talk to each other in disparaging or demeaning ways, if they fail to provide information about their activities, or if they distort or selectively communicate information.

Effective communication occurs when all participants:

- Listen attentively to each other
- Accept and act upon what is said
- Can understand what has been said
- Are truthful and sincere
- Act in socially and culturally appropriate ways
- Regularly advise others about what is happening

Participation

When people participate actively in research tasks their worth is acknowledged and high levels of personal investment—resources, time, and emotion—often result. Active participation is very empowering, especially for people who have a poor self-image. Sometimes people may commence with quite simple tasks, taking on increasingly complex activities as their confidence increases. Although this sometimes requires more time and considerable patience on the part of research facilitators, the long-term benefits easily outweigh the initial outlay of time and effort.

Participation is most effective when it:

- Enables significant levels of active involvement
- Enables people to perform significant tasks
- Provides support for people as they learn to act for themselves
- Encourages plans and activities that people are able to accomplish themselves
- Deals personally with people rather than with their representatives or agent

Inclusion

In professional life, there is often pressure to find short-term solutions to complex problems, providing practitioners and/or administrators with the temptation to find superficial and limited solutions. Usually, these actions fail to take into account many of the factors contributing to the problem or to include people who are an integral part of the context.

Inclusion requires participants to:

- Involve all relevant groups and individuals whose lives are affected by the issue investigated
- Take account of all relevant issues affecting the research question
- Cooperate with related groups, agencies, and organizations when necessary
- Ensure that all relevant groups benefit from activities

Conclusion

As health professionals engage in participatory action research with clients, colleagues, and/or members of the community, they will meet many obstacles that threaten to frustrate the harmonious resolution of the problems and issues they are investigating. By enacting the working principles of action research that speak to issues of relationship, communication, inclusion, and participation, they maximize the possibility of engaging whole-hearted support and engagement of the people involved. Action research engages technical routines of inquiry, but must also take into account the human dimensions of the process to acquire the greatest benefit for the clients, patients, and consumers of health care programs and services.

SUMMARY

This chapter describes procedures for initiating a study:

Setting the stage **to create a productive research environment by taking into account people's feelings of** *pride, dignity, identity,* **and** *responsibility.*

Research planning and design **involves** *focusing* **the study,** *framing* **it by delimiting the scope of the inquiry, engaging in a prelim-inary,** *literature review, sampling*—**selecting study participants, and establishing procedures for gathering and analyzing data.**

Research ethics **must be established to ensure** *confidentiality* **and duty of** *care.* **Formal institutional** *protocols* **for approval should be enacted and** *informed consent* **obtained from participants.**

Validty **of the study should also be established, research procedures ensuring that the quality and** *trustworthiness* **of the study is credible, transferable, dependable, and confirmable.**

Working principles **of** *relationships, communication, participation,* **and** *inclusion* **provide the means to heighten the degree of engagement of participants.**

Gathering Data: Sources of Information

RESEARCH DESIGN	DATA GATHERING	DATA ANALYSIS	COMMUNICATION	ACTION
			WRITING REPORTS	CREATING SOLUTIONS
INITIATING A STUDY	CAPTURING STAKEHOLDER EXPERIENCES AND PERSPECTIVES	IDENTIFYING KEY FEATURES OF EXPERIENCE	Reports Ethnographies Biographies	Care plans
Setting the stage				Case managment
Focusing and framing	Interviewing	Analyzing epiphanies and illuminative experiences	PRESENTATIONS AND PERFORMANCES	Problem-solving
Literature review	Observing			
Stakeholders	Reviewing artifacts	Categorizing and coding	Presentations Drama Poetry	Enhancing practices
Data sources	Reviewing literature	Enhancing analysis	Song Dance Art	Evaluation
Ethics			Video Multimedia	Health promotion
Validity		Constructing category frameworks		Community development
				Professional development
				Strategic planning

Contents of This Chapter

Chapter 3 described the first phase of inquiry in which participants focus their investigation and design on a valid and ethical research process. This chapter presents the first steps of that investigation, describing procedures for systematically accumulating information that will contribute to extended understanding of the issue investigated. It provides details of:

- The *purposes* for gathering information
- Procedures for *interviewing* participants
- Procedures for *observing* settings and events
- Procedures for reviewing *artifacts*—records, documents, and materials
- Procedures for incorporating *statistical and numerical data*, including those obtained from *surveys*
- Procedures for reviewing the *literature*

Building a Picture: Gathering Information

The first movement through the Look-Think-Act research cycle provided preliminary information from which participants defined the research problem and question
and a plan for enacting the investigation. During the next iteration of the cycle, both
the research facilitators and other participants begin to build a picture of the problem they are investigating, first focusing on the Look step by gathering information
from a variety of sources (see Figure 4.1). Ultimately, this information will be used
to develop detailed accounts that clarify and extend their understanding of the acts,
activities, events, purposes, and emotions comprising people's everyday lives.

Qualitative, interpretive processes of inquiry seek to understand the experience
of interacting individuals. When we work with clients or patients who appear igno-
rant of factors affecting their health, people who seem reluctant to engage with qualified health professionals, or those who are obviously incapable of managing their
health, we wonder, "What is happening for this person? What is their experience?
What is their understanding of the situation?" Action research seeks an understanding of the experience and perspective of individual clients or patients and other
stakeholders—parents, friends and relatives, supervisors, employers, and other significant actors.

In action research, **interviews** are the principle means of understanding
people's experiences and perspectives. Information is also gathered by systematic
observation of settings and events, **reviewing relevant documents** and
records, and examining related **materials** and **equipment.** Numerical and statistical information may complement other data. Relevant literature—including academic research reports, professional publications, or official reports—may further

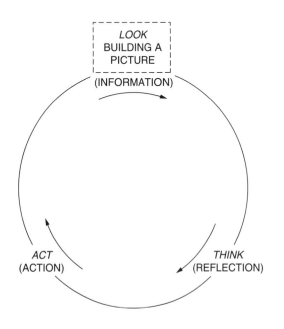

Figure 4.1
Obtaining Information
in Action Research

Medical sociology consistently presents accounts of "modern," well-equipped health clinics in non-Western or inner-urban settings that local people are reluctant to use. Explanations for the non-utilization of services include: clinics demanding hard currency for services in a community where the norm is for goods and services to be bartered; the scheduled clinic hours coinciding with the only period in the day when paid work is available for either women or men; previous experiences of non-consensual procedures performed by clinic staff; and situations where clinic staff belong to a group in the community with whom members of other groups are unwilling to interact. In these instances, clinics and their associated services often have been developed without engaging in the necessary research to understand how the facilities and services might be set up to operate effectively. Often, clinic staff explain such situations as a lack of gratitude or a persistence of belief in traditional medicines by local people, assuming their own knowledge and experience is a sufficient basis for making decisions about building and operating a clinic. There is a clear need, in these types of contexts, for the professionals concerned to engage local knowledge to ensure that desired health and medical outcomes are achievable.

illuminate the issue investigated. Each of these types of information—records of interviews, observations, and reviews of documents, artifacts, and literature—has the potential to increase the power and scope of the research process. If we not only listen to people describe and interpret their experience, but observe and participate in events, and read reports of those or similar events, then we enrich the research process. This **triangulation** of data adds depth and rigor to the research process.

Interviewing: Guided Conversations

Interviews enable participants to describe their situation and reveal their own interpretation of issues investigated. They enable participants to "enter the world" of the person interviewed and to understand events from their perspective (Denzin, 1997; Spradley, 1979a; Spradley & McCurdy, 1972). Interviews not only provide a record of interviewee views and perspectives, but also symbolically recognize the legitimacy of their point of view. They are the principal means by which we are able to "hear the voice of the other" and incorporate their perspective into the inquiry process. Interviews also provide opportunities for participants to revisit and reflect on events in their lives, and in so doing, extend their understanding of their own experience. This double hermeneutic—meaning-making process—serves as the principal powerhouse of the research process, enabling all participants to extend their understanding of their own and others' experience.

Interviewing is best accomplished as a sociable series of events, not unlike a conversation between friends where the easy exchange of information takes place in a comfortable, friendly environment. Although some people envisage interviewing as a form of authentic dialogue, we need to be wary of the way this dialogue emerges. When interviewers engage in exchanges of information or experience, as in a normal conversation, they unwittingly inscribe their own sets of meanings onto the dialogue, constructing descriptions and interpretations that distort the experience or perspective of the participant interviewed. The following protocols provide ways to engage the interview process comfortably, ethically, and productively.

A wide range of literature provides information about interviewing (e.g., Chirban, 1996; Holstein & Gubrium, 1995; Kvale, 1996; McCracken, 1988; Rubin & Rubin, 1995). Researchers should use these materials selectively, however, since some interview techniques are used for clinical or hypothesis testing processes not suited to the purposes of action research. The key issue guiding selection of technique is whether it is used to reveal the perspective of the participant or whether it focuses on revealing specified types of information.

Initiating Interviews: Establishing Relationships of Trust

Initial stages of the interview process can be a little uncomfortable for both interviewer and interviewee, and the interviewer must establish a relationship of trust in order to enable the interviewee to feel able to reveal their experience, either to a stranger or a colleague. Chapter 3 suggests using initial contacts with people to inform them of the issue being studied and to explore the possibility that they might participate. The researcher:

- Identifies themselves
- Identifies the issue of interest
- Asks permission to talk about that issue
- Negotiates a convenient time and place to meet

The actual conversation may sound something like:

Hi! I'm Ernie Stringer. The director says he's informed the staff I'd be working here. I've been asked to help them explore ways of improving patient adherence to care plans. I'd like to hear your views about that. Could we set up a time to talk? I'd need about half an hour of your time.

The primary consideration in interviewing is for the interviewee to feel comfortable and safe talking with the interviewer. Interviews should be initiated in ways appropriate to the people and setting that enable respondents to feel in control of the situation—to make them feel they are not being put upon. Provide them with opportunities to determine both the time and place of interviews, and ask them to suggest places to meet where they are comfortable. A clinic or office may not be the best place to interview clients—the site itself having possible negative connotations negatively affecting a participant's state of mind. Research is a sociable process and should be treated as such. According to the circumstances, people may be comfortable in their own homes, in cafés or fast food outlets, or in a park or other public place. A meeting over coffee enables interviewer and interviewee to chat about general events and establish a conversational tone in their interactions. This provides a context to move easily to the issue of interest.

Initiating interviews sometimes is a sensitive process. Initially, you might manage with short chats in hallways and lounges, which open possibilities for more extended conversations (interviews). It is important to keep these initial occasions low key and informal so people feel they are not being imposed upon. After an initial interaction, you might indicate your desire to have them speak at greater length about issues arising in your conversation. Let them know the focus of your interests and that you are interested in their perspective. "This has been interesting, Jack. I'd like to be able to explore this issue further. Could we meet somewhere and continue this conversation?" This provides a context for commencing more in-depth conversations that provide the basis for a continuing research relationship.

Questioning Techniques

Spradley (1979a) provides a useful framework of questions derived from his attempts to elicit natural structures of meaning used by people to describe and organize their social worlds. His essentially ethnographic methodology suggests the use of neutral, non-leading questions that minimize the extent to which participant responses will be governed by frameworks of meaning inadvertently imposed by the researcher. A modified form of this framework provides the means to engage in extended interviews revealing detailed descriptions of events and interactions in participants' lives and providing opportunities to explore significant issues in depth in their own terms.

A major problem with the interview process is that researcher perceptions, perspectives, interests, and agendas easily flavor questions when the major purpose of the process is to obtain interviewee perspectives. Common approaches to interviewing based on extended lists of pre-defined, highly structured questions, therefore, are inappropriate for the purpose of this type of research. Ethnographic interviews are quite different from questionnaires that frame the issue in terms making sense to the researcher, often focusing on technical/professional concepts, agendas, procedures, or practices. This detracts from the ability of participants to define, describe, and interpret experiences in their own terms, and can sometimes alienate audiences central to the study.

The following questioning schema is based on that developed by Spradley (1979a).

Phase One: Grand Tour Questions

An action research interview begins with one general grand tour question taking the form:

"Tell me about . . . ." "Tell me about your illness." "Tell me about the clinic." Though there are many extensions from this fundamental query, the simple framing enables respondents to describe, frame, and interpret events, issues, and other phenomena in their own terms. The grand tour question is not asked in bald isolation, but emerges contextually when sufficient rapport has been established. It is also necessary to *frame* or contextualize the question.

*There are a number of clients concerned about [treatments at this clinic]. Last time we talked you spoke briefly about this issue. Could you **tell me about** [your experience of treatment here]?*

Often, it is best to contextualize the issue by starting with a more general question:

*Last time we spoke of treatments at this clinic. I'm not very familiar with this clinic. Could you **tell me about** the clinic.*

In most cases, people are able to talk at length on an issue about which they are concerned. It merely requires a listener with an attentive attitude to enable them to engage in an extended discourse, sometimes encouraged by prompts (see the following) to extend their descriptions. In some instances, however, participants may be unable to answer such a general question, tempting the researcher to insert more specific questions that undermine the intent of the research process. Spradley (1979a) suggests alternative ways of asking grand tour questions when respondents are able only to give limited responses to the more general question:

- **Typical** grand tour questions, enabling respondents to talk of ways events usually occur (e.g., How does treatment usually occur? Describe a typical treatment session.)
- **Specific** grand tour questions, which focus on particular events or times (e.g., Can you tell me about yesterday's treatment session? Describe what happened the last time?)
- **A guided tour** question is a request for an actual tour that allows participants to show researchers (and, where possible, other stakeholders) around sites associated with the issue investigated (e.g., Could you show me around the clinic?) As they walk around the clinic, participants may explain details about the people and activities involved in each part of the setting. Researchers may use **mini-tour** or **prompt** questions (see the following box) to extend the descriptions provided (e.g., Tell me more about what happens in this part of the clinic. Can you tell me more about the nurses/physician/intern you've mentioned?).
- **A task-related** grand tour question aids in description (e.g., Could you draw me a map of the clinic?). Maps are often very instructive and provide opportunities for extensive description and questioning. You can also ask participants to demonstrate how things are done (e.g., Can you show me how you undertake your treatment? Can you show me how the equipment works?).

Grand tour questions comprise ways of initiating participant descriptions of their experience. Information acquired in this way provides the basis for more extended descriptions, elicited by similar types of questions, but emerging from ideas, agendas, concepts, and meanings implicit in the respondents' own descriptions.

Novice researchers sometimes find interviewing an uncomfortable experience. The process of working through structured questioning processes often feels awkward and unnatural, and they tend to fall back on conversation as a means of engaging participants. Practice and experience, however, show how it is possible for interview questions to freely and easily construct a conversation. In the best formulation, questions should emerge in a friendly, informal manner, echoing informal talk amongst friends—"What's happening? What's up? What's going on?"

Novice researchers should prepare for interviewing processes by memorizing the forms of questioning described herein and practicing mock interviews with friends and colleagues. Such role plays can assist interviewers to translate seemingly formal interview formats into conversational language of participating groups. Like any set of skills, practice may not make perfect, but it certainly increases effectiveness.

An interesting outcome of the acquisition of these questioning skills is their more general application to health contexts. Health practitioners will find them wonderful tools for client interviews, and administrators will find them useful in refining aspects of their managerial work—consultation, planning, leadership, and organization. A community health nurse wrote of this work in a message to a colleague:

> *Spradley's format is very helpful when I apply it to talking with my patients. I use the visual cues, have them write stuff out on paper, make drawings, maps of the clinic. The work is shared. We physically walk the area—a guided tour. I first thought the idea was dumb, but it's a great success. It's engaged, it's shared, we are walking together. The movement stops the tape in the head. The experience is shared. It's generative.*

Phase Two: Extending the Interview—Mini-Tour Questions

Interviews emerge and expand from responses to initial grand tour questions. As people respond to the initial grand tour questions, a number of details begin to emerge, revealing events, activities, issues, concerns, and so on, that comprise their experience and perspective. Sometimes the information is limited or somewhat superficial and interviewers need to probe further to enable the respondent to dig deeper into their experience. At this stage, further questions emerge from concepts, issues, and ideas embedded in respondent answers to the first grand tour questions (Figure 4.2). The interviewer asks **mini-tour** questions, uses the concepts and language of the respondent, and enables them to extend their responses in their own terms.

Mini-tour questions are similar in form to the general, typical, specific, guided, and task-related grand tour questions, but the focus of the questions is derived from information revealed in initial responses. They take the form:

> *"You talked about client visits. Can you tell me more about client visits?"*
> Or *"Tell me what you usually do during a client visit?"*
> Or *"Tell me what happened during your last client visit?"*
> Or *"Can you show me your clinic, and tell me what happens there during a client visit?"*
> Or *"Can you show me or demonstrate what you do during a patient visit?"*

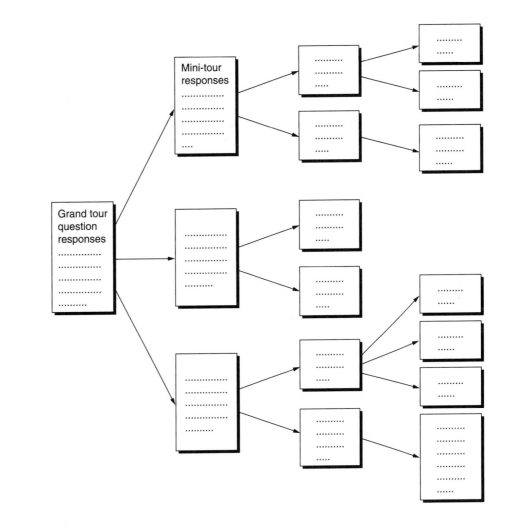

Figure 4.2
Mini-Tour
Questioning
Processes

Mini-tour questions can also be aimed particularly at revealing meanings embedded in the language of participant groups:

> *"Earlier you talked about being a 'support' to the client. Tell me more about being a 'support.'"*
> Or *". . . you talked about having to 'hang' in the waiting room after you have seen the physician. Tell me more about 'hanging.'"*
> Or *". . . you mentioned that you encourage the clients to 'take control of their lives.' Tell me more about clients 'taking control of their lives.'"*
> Or *". . . you mentioned that you encourage the clients to 'take control of their lives.' Can you tell me about a client who has 'taken control of their life?'"*

Responses to these questions may lead to further mini-tour questions, which can eventually provide extended, detailed descriptions of the issues and contexts investigated.

Extending Participant Responses: Prompt Questions

Further information may be acquired through the skilful use of prompts, enabling participants to reveal more details of the phenomena they are discussing:

- **Extension** questions (e.g., Tell me more about. . . . Is there anything else you can tell me about? What else?)
- **Encouragement** comments/questions (e.g., Go on Yes? Uh-huh? Mmmm?)
- **Example** questions (e.g., Can you give me an example of how you usually begin a consultation?)

Prompt questions are not designed to elicit particular types of information the interviewer might see as desirable, but merely to enable the interviewee to think more closely about events or perspectives described.

As interviews progress, research facilitators may be presented with viewpoints that appear limited, biased, wrong, or potentially harmful. They should, however, not attempt to extend the participants' responses by suggesting appropriate responses—"Don't you think that . . . ," and definitely must avoid discussion or debate about information presented. Interviewers should also avoid criticizing the perspective presented or suggesting alternative acceptable viewpoints. Acceptance of diverse viewpoints is a prime directive in action research, even when those perspectives conflict dramatically with those of other research participants. Challenges to particular viewpoints will occur naturally as differing perspectives are presented in more public arenas. The task at this stage is to grasp a person's point of view and to realize their vision of their world (Malinowski, 1922/1961). A wide range of literature provides information about interviewing (Chirban 1996; Holstein & Gubrium, 1995; Kvale, 1996; McCracken, 1988; Rubin & Rubin, 1995), though researchers should be selective—some interview techniques are not suited to the purposes of action research. The defining criterion for selecting a particular technique is the extent to which it enables the perspective, language, and concepts of the interviewee to drive the interview process.

In the course of work with senior government department managers, my Aboriginal colleagues and I sometimes faced people whose perspectives were fundamentally racist. I would converse with them with barely controlled rage, fuming at the insensitive nature of their remarks. On one occasion, an Aboriginal colleague later said, "Take it easy, Stringer. He doesn't understand," to which I responded, "How do you stand it?" He looked at me quizzically and said, "You just get used to it." In many of these situations, we were able to engage in productive work with these departments that, in the longer term, sensitized the people with whom we had been speaking to their inappropriate behavior and/or perspectives. I learned at that time that immediate confrontation is not always an appropriate response to inappropriate speech or behavior.

Prolonged Engagement

The intent of action research is to help people develop new understandings of issues or problems. Merely asking them to "explain" why and how the issue affects them often elicits merely taken-for-granted responses or perspectives that reproduce superficial understandings. Such responses provide little basis for revealing implicit meanings and underlying features of their experience. Interview processes should give people the opportunity to carefully reflect on their experience, examining how events and issues are embedded in the complexity of events that comprise their everyday life.

The questioning techniques described previously help facilitate this descriptive process, but are only effective if sufficient time is allocated to enable participants to explore the issue in depth. While some problems or issues may require relatively small investments of time, larger or long-standing issues often require prolonged periods of reflection and analysis. While a single 15–20 minute interview may suffice for a simple issue, significant issues may require multiple interviews of 30–60 minutes in duration, enabling participants to explore issues in depth, engaging the multiple dimensions of their experience and, in the process, extending their understanding of the complexity of the issues they face.

Repeat interviews, therefore, are an essential feature of good qualitative research. They not only enable participants to reflect on issues more extensively, but provide opportunities to review and extend information previously acquired. Extended engagement suggests the need for a significant time commitment and repeated interaction with or between research participants. Merely being in the context is not sufficient—one must be engaged in systematic inquiry required to *re-search* an issue in context.

When I queried the apparently inadequate interview processes of one researcher, she replied, "Oh, I was working with those nurses for months." Unfortunately, the intensive nature of the clinical work in which the nurses and researcher were engaged provided little opportunity for them to discuss the nature of their experience. Most of their attention was focused on the provision of care and technical issues related to the project. The single 15-minute interview for each nurse was an inadequate vehicle for revealing the complex nature of their experience, providing only superficial comments that were uninformative and uninspiring.

Recording Information

Although action research processes often are informal, especially in small-scale or localized projects, it is important to keep a record of information acquired. This is especially important when different groups are involved, where personality differences are likely to create discord, or where sensitive issues are investigated. Participants acquire a degree of safety knowing their perspectives are not forgotten or distorted over time. For reasons of accuracy and harmony, an ongoing record of information is a central feature of research. Field notes and tape recordings provide the two major forms of recording information, though increasing use is being made of video recording.

On numerous occasions, I have been engaged in action research projects that threatened to be disrupted by disputes about things people had said or decisions that had been made. Referring back to the recorded data and reading the actual words people had used usually restores order when disputes threaten to erupt. In numerous instances, a mollified participant has acknowledged his or her error by saying, "Did I say that?" or "I forgot that we'd decided that."

Field Notes

Verbatim record Wherever possible, interviewers should make an immediate record of responses. You should ask the respondent's permission to do so before the interview, or in some cases, after the first few minutes, when the person has commenced talking. You might say, "This is very interesting. Do you mind if I take notes as you talk?" Handwritten field notes provide the means to obtain a written verbatim record of people's actual words. This requires researchers to record what is *actually said* by the person being interviewed, rather than a condensed or "tidied up" version. It is a "warts and all" procedure, where colloquialisms, incorrect grammar, or even blatantly incorrect information are precisely recorded. Scribes recording information need to be wary of paraphrasing or abstracting, since this defeats the purpose of interviewing (i.e., capturing the voice of participants and describing things as they would describe them). At later stages of the interview (see member checking, which follows), the interviewee will have opportunities to correct or add to the information given.

The following example is a record of an interview with a nurse:

Interviewer: Some nurses have told me they'd like greater family participation in the preparation of care plans. Can you tell me what you think of this idea?

Nurse: Well, family members should feel they are part of the siuation. We could provide, like, information for family members on things like handling equipment, using medication, you know . . .

It would help people to have skills to assist their family, especially those who're struggling. They could be offered information sessions, like caring skills, how to develop good health habits. It'd be low pressure, low key. You could have staff volunteers with special skills, special expertise.

It helps establish good relationships with families and patients. Give them greater ability to communicate about care procedures. They'd be able to talk more easily about their family members' care.

Interviewer: Are their other ways to increase family participation?

Nurse: I like having partners or parents who can guide and help patients, but not do what has to be done for them. Some people help, but they end up doing things themselves. That's not on. But if they help the patients with their care plan, it's a great help to me.

A handwritten record requires practice in writing at speed and the concomitant development of personal "shorthand" writing protocols— "&" for "and," "w/" for "with," "t" for "the," "g" for "ing," missing consonants (e.g., writg or wrtg for writing), and so on. It takes practice, but is essential if researchers are to record the respondent's actual words. Sometimes, it may be necessary to ask the person interviewed to repeat information, or to pause momentarily so the interviewee can catch up on their notes.

Member checking   Once an interview has finished, the interviewer should read back the notes giving the respondent an opportunity to confirm the accuracy of the notes or to extend or clarify information. In some cases, it may also be possible to identify key features of the interview to use in data analysis (see Chapter 5: Analyzing Data). Some people type their notes and have the respondent read it to check for accuracy. It may also be appropriate, in some instances, to provide a copy of the field notes to the respondent for their own information.

Tape Recorders

Using a tape recorder has the advantage of allowing the researcher to acquire a detailed and accurate account of an interview. Researchers acquire large quantities of information from multiple sources, so a careful record of tapes should be maintained, noting on each tape the person, place, times, and date of the interview.

Tape recordings have a number of disadvantages, however, and researchers should carefully weigh the merits of this technology. Technical difficulties with equipment may result in loss of data and can damage rapport with respondents. People sometimes find it difficult to talk freely in the presence of a recording device, especially when sensitive issues are discussed. A researcher may need to wait until a reasonable degree of rapport has been established before introducing the possibility of using a tape recorder. When using a recorder, the researcher should be prepared to stop the tape to allow respondents to speak "off the record" if they show signs of discomfort.

The sheer volume of material obtained through tape recording also may inhibit the steady progress of a research process. Researchers should be wary of accumulating tapes for later transcribing. Frequently, this becomes a lengthy and tedious process that can detract from the power of the research, particularly when emergent issues within an interview are relegated to the archive, albeit temporarily, rather than sparking a new branch of investigation. If tape recordings are used, they should be transcribed immediately so that relevant information may become available to participants. This is particularly useful when contentious or sensitive issues are explored, since a person's own words may help resolve potentially inflammatory situations.

Using Focus Groups to Gather Data

In recent years, focus groups have emerged as a useful way to engage people in processes of investigation. They enable research participants to share information and experiences that "trigger" new ideas or insights, and provide greater insight into events and activities. A focus group may be envisioned as a group interview with questions providing a stimulus for capturing people's experiences and perspectives. It provides the means for including relatively large numbers of people in a research process, an important consideration in larger projects.

Joint processes of collaborative description and analysis considerably enhance the power of a research process. Focus groups provide the context for people to identify and name shared categories of experience or to identify different ways they have interpreted events. Individual interviews followed by focus group exploration provide a context for participants to share information and extend their understanding of issues.

Action research, therefore, increases in power when undertaken as a *participatory* process that fosters the interactive engagement of participants. The power increases exponentially when such participatory processes become collaborative and when respondents begin to ask questions of other respondents and the research facilitator. By working together, sharing ideas, and exploring their collective experience and perspectives, the productive, creative, and innovative possibilities of action research emerge strongly.

A cyclical process of investigation emerges, depicted in the concept map of Figure 4.3. Interviews lead to individual accounts that are shared and then formulated into joint accounts that record both commonalities and divergences of experience and perspective.

When we bring diverse groups together, however, we need to carefully manage the dynamics of interaction and discussion to ensure the productive operation of focus groups. Too easily, they sometimes degenerate into "gab-fests" or "slinging matches" where unfocused discussions or argumentative interchanges damage the harmonious qualities characteristic of good action research. Helpful literature for facilitating focus groups includes Barbour and Kitzinger (1998), Morgan (1997a, 1997b), Morgan and Krueger (1997), Krueger (1994, 1997a, 1997b), Krueger and Casey (2000), and Greenbaum (2000).

Bringing People Together

To initiate focus group explorations, the research facilitator should seek opportunities to convene forums where participants can discuss issues of common interest. "I've spoken with a number of people about this issue and some of them have similar

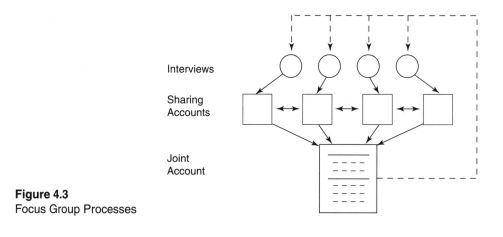

Figure 4.3
Focus Group Processes

views to yourself. Would you be willing to meet with them to talk about the issues you've raised?" Or "As you know, I've been speaking with other nurses, and some are concerned about . . . Would you attend a meeting with people like Janet Jones, Bill Rochon, and Maria Garcia to discuss this issue?"

As with interviews, the time and the place must be conducive to the process. People should have adequate time to explore the issue and should be in a place where they are comfortable and feel they can express their views and experiences freely. A rushed meeting during a coffee break or in a cafeteria where others can overhear is likely to limit the information shared and is unlikely to generate the positive working relationships required. These issues are especially important when working with clients or their families. As with interviews, meetings away from clinics or formal settings may be more conducive to the production of an easy and communicative atmosphere, providing the basis for ongoing development of productive action research processes.

The use of focus groups at meetings is especially productive because they provide opportunities for a large number of individuals to share their perceptions and experiences. The size of groups is important, with four to six people being the optimal number for enabling everyone to participate effectively.

Focus groups can be used in contexts large and small. When working with staff from a community health training program to facilitate an internal review of curriculum implementation, I interviewed each staff member separately. I then wrote a short report revealing the issues that emerged from these interactions. After staff had read the report, I facilitated a focus group meeting enabling them to clarify issues in the report and to identify and prioritize issues on which they wished to take action. Because it was a small work unit, we were able to complete this process within a week.

On another occasion, I worked with a group of community health workers and administrators at a small rural health center who were concerned about the use of alcohol in the community and the associated trauma presented at the clinic. The community health workers were interested in community perceptions of the issue, but were conscious of the difficulty of approaching households where alcohol use was known to be high. After experimenting with ways to approach households using role-play methods, the community health workers presented themselves to households as professionals concerned with suffering in the community and seeking community perceptions about the suffering caused by alcohol. After analyzing the interview data, the health workers presented the results at a community meeting where the issues were ascribed different priorities. Over a period of six months, health workers and community members met to seek further information, clarify concerns, and develop and implement action plans to address the issues.

Focus Group Processes

Focus group sessions should be carefully planned and facilitated to ensure the productive use of time. Poorly prepared groups too easily degenerate into gossip sessions to be dominated by a forceful person, or to create antagonisms derived from intemperate debates. The following steps provide a basic procedure for running focus groups:

1. Set ground rules
   - Each person should have opportunities to express their perspective
   - All perspectives should be accepted nonjudgmentally
   - And so on.
2. Provide clear guidance
   - Provide and display focus questions
   - Designate a time frame for each section/question
3. Designate a facilitator for each group to
   - Ensure each person has an equal chance to talk
   - Keep discussions on track
   - Monitor times
4. Record group talk in each group
   - Designate a person to record proceedings
   - Record detail of each person's contribution, using their own words
   - Where appropriate, each group should summarize their discussions, identifying and recording key features of participant experiences, and significant issues or problems
5. Feedback and clarification
   - Bring groups together, ensuring adequate time is available for feedback and discussion
   - Have each group present the summary of their discussions
   - Provide opportunities for individuals within each group to extend or clarify points presented
   - The facilitator should ask questions of each group designed to have them clarify and extend their contribution
   - Ensure that new information emerging from this process is recorded
6. Analyze combined information
   - Identify common features across groups
   - Identify divergent issues or perspectives
   - Rank issues in order of priority
7. What next: A plan for action
   - Define what is to happen next: What actions are to be taken, who will be responsible for them, where and when they will be done, what resources are required, and who will organize these actions
   - Designate a person to monitor these actions
   - Designate a time and place to meet again to review progress

These seemingly bland procedures mask the exciting and rewarding possibilities emerging from dialogue, discussion, and personal interactions common in these types of process. The benefits gained by providing participants with the space and time to engage in open dialogue on issues about which they are deeply concerned include increased clarity and understanding, and the development of productive personal relationships so important to the effective enactment of action research.

Focus Questions

The major purpose of these types of sessions is to provide people with opportunities to describe and reflect on their own experiences and perspectives. A general statement by the facilitator contextualizing and framing the issue should be followed by a series of *focus questions* similar in format to those provided for individual interviews.

Grand tour questions enable people to express their experience and perspectives in their own terms: "We're meeting today to think about ways we might more effectively link with potential clients in our community. I'd like to give you time, initially, to talk about ways you currently link with potential clients, then extend our discussions from there. Please focus initially on the first question 'How do I link currently with families?'"

Mini-tour questions As people explore these issues, further questions may emerge from issues arising in their discussion. "There's not enough time," "There are some potential clients who don't wish to make contact," and so on. These statements are reframed in question form and become the subject for further sharing of information: "What are the different ways we currently make time to link with potential clients?" "What are the ways we currently link with clients who don't want to make contact?" The sharing of information in this way not only enables people to benefit from each other's experience, but also provides possibilities for directly formulating solutions to issues as they emerge.

Guided tour questions Focus groups may engage in a guided tour, in which people tour a clinic, hospital, or health facility, sharing their experiences or perspectives of events related to those environments.

Task-related questions Groups may also benefit from task-related questions, so that members are able to demonstrate how they go about achieving some purpose: "Could you show us how you organize the lessons you've been talking about?" "Could you show the group how you conduct an initial interview with a client?" "Could you demonstrate how you show clients how to use this piece of equipment?" Having people express their perspective artistically or visually can sometimes provide very evocative understandings of their experience, and maps and diagrams may be similarly productive. Facilitators may ask people, either individually or as a group, to draw a picture, a map, or a diagram illustrating their experience of the issue on which they are focused. These productions then become the focus for further discussions extending people's understanding of participant experiences and perspectives.

The use of activities and physical demonstrations or representations of experience are well known techniques in primary health care and health promotion and have been documented in the literature on Participatory Rural Appraisal (Chambers, 1992; Mascarenhas, 1992). Participants use drama, diagrams, maps, models, inscriptions, natural materials, and objects to represent their experience, rank preferences, draw

comparisons about wealth and well-being, or represent timelines and seasonal varia-
tions. Providing the means for participants to represent their experience in a variety of
media is crucial when working in situations where diverse cultural traditions operate.

Facilitators should ensure that each group keeps an ongoing record of their discussion. This may take the form of notes, recorded by a volunteer in the group, but
sometimes may be recorded in summary form on charts. Where multiple groups are
engaged in discussions, a plenary session should provide opportunities for participants to share the results of their exploration.

Overview: Interviews and Focus Groups

Interviews and focus groups provide the principal entry into an action research
process. They provide the means for all stakeholders to reveal their experience and
to extend and explore their understanding of the issues investigated. Through continued questioning, participants seek to uncover the often-unquestioned assumptions embedded in their world-views and to make explicit the taken-for-granted
knowledge inscribed in their everyday activities. Thus, they seek greater clarity in
understanding the complexities of the situation and provide the groundwork for developing solutions to the problems they encounter. Interviews, however, are not the
sole means of acquiring information. As the following sections describe, participants
can extend their understanding by careful observation and by reviewing information
from other sources.

Participant Observation

The principal purpose of observation is to familiarize research participants with the
context in which issues and events are played out, or to provide participants with
opportunities to stand back from their everyday activities and observe purposefully
as events unfold. Careful observation enables participants to "build a picture" of the
context and the activities and events within it, revealing details of the setting as
well as the mundane, routine activities comprising the life-world of clients, colleagues, and the community. Sometimes, however, observation is revelatory, providing keen insights or illuminating important but taken-for-granted features of the
context.

Observation in action research is very different from the highly structured
types of observation required in experimental research, where the researcher
records the frequency of specific types of behavior, acts, or events using a highly
structured observation schedule. Participant observation in action research is
much less structured and more open-ended, its purpose being to provide more detailed descriptions of people's actions and the context in which they occur. Participant observation seeks a deeper level of understanding through extended
immersion in the context and interaction with associated people and events
within it.

As with interviewing, observation requires focus so that relevant features of the
scene are recorded. Spradley (1979b) suggests that observations should always be
accompanied or preceded by relevant questions for this purpose. A research facili-

tator may ask participants for a guided tour, while holding in mind the underlying question—"What do I need to know about this place to understand the issue investigated? Tell me about this clinic (your family, community, etc.)." Participant observations will be enriched as they focus on:

- **People:** clients, family members, administrators, allied and support staff, and so on
- **Places:** reception rooms, consulting rooms, offices, client homes, community contexts, locations of activities and events, and physical layouts
- **Acts:** single actions that people take (e.g., a nurse consoling a client)
- **Activities:** a set of related acts (e.g., a physician engaging in a consultation)
- **Events:** a set of related activities (e.g., a community health nurse undertaking a home visit)
- **Objects:** buildings, furniture, equipment, instruments, medication, and so on
- **Purposes:** what people are trying to accomplish
- **Time:** times, frequency, duration, and sequencing of events and activities
- **Feelings:** emotional orientations and responses to people, events, activities, and so on

Working with participants in this way enables research facilitators to check the veracity of their own observations. This is an important issue—it is all too easy for an outside researcher to focus on irrelevant issues or to misinterpret events.

In an inquiry into the practice of community health nurses, I carefully recorded features of the households they visited. I observed the decorations and family photographs on the wall, the style of the furniture, the activities of the grandchildren, and the interaction amongst family members. When these reports were presented back to the nurses, they were able to elaborate on taken-for-granted features of the context that had significant impact on their work. For example, they described how clients were affected by the presence and behavior of children at consultations in the home, and also focused on the poverty evident in households, both features of the situation I had failed to note in my own observations.

Recording Observations

Field Notes

Researchers should record their observations in field notes that provide ongoing records of important acts, activities, and events. Field notes comprise the vital repository of data that will both guide further inquiry and provide the material from which research outcomes will emerge. Field notes enable researchers to record detailed descriptions of actual places and events as they observe the settings and events in which participants carry out their daily activities. While it is not always possible to record field notes immediately, observers should record events as soon as possible after the events occur.

The task may appear quite daunting as any context contains huge amounts of information that could be recorded. As indicated previously, researchers should record that information needed to understand the *context* of the issue investigated, using the provided framework as a guide (people, places, events, etc.). The recorded information provides material that will later be used to provide descriptions of the context of the research or of events and activities.

Hand-drawn maps or pictures may supplement written descriptions to provide increased clarity. A map of a clinic, hospital, or neighborhood, for instance, provides a pictorial representation that may be later used to provide increased understanding and clarity. Observers may "set up" their observations by describing and drawing the setting and recording pertinent events and activities as they occur over a period of time, then member checking to ensure appropriate renditions of both setting and events.

Tape Recording

Tape recorded information provides a detailed recording of all that is said in a given situation. This type of record provides clear evidence of what is actually said by participants and can help research participants describe and clarify recorded events. Tape-recording of naturally occurring conversations enables researchers to check the veracity of their observations and analysis. It also provides the means to ensure that language and concepts used in analysis and reporting match those of the participants.

On one particular occasion during fieldwork, I became acutely conscious of the way I had skewed interpretation of events. On this occasion, as is evident in the transcript below, I was challenged directly by the person concerned,

Bill: "What you have been saying is that the problem, then, is that people have to pay and that a lot of people *don't want to pay*. Is that right?. . . "
June: "Quite often *they haven't got money.*"
Bill: "Yeah."
June: "Not that they *don't want to pay.*"
Bill: "Oh no—but I mean—yeah, they don't have money or whatever."

Photographs

Photographs provide a graphic record that enables later audiences to more clearly visualize settings and events. Photographs are a particularly useful means of stimulating discussion during focus groups and may provide the basis for focusing and/or extending interviews. A mini-tour question—"Tell me what's happening in this photograph"—can provide richly detailed descriptions, an especially useful process when working with children or elderly clients. Photographs may also be used to enhance reports presented to participants or to other research audiences.

Video Recording

Video equipment is also an important research resource. Written descriptions are necessarily limited, being highly dependant on the skills of the writer and often providing inadequate and incomplete understanding of events and contexts. Video recording has the advantage of making the scene immediately available to viewers, providing a far greater depth of understanding of the acts, activities, events, interactions, behaviors, and the nature of the context. While limited by the focusing mechanisms of the photographer, extended video recordings can reveal highly informative pictures easily viewed by large audiences.

Careful consideration needs to be given to the specific settings and events to be recorded. Schouten and Watling (1997) suggest a process by which participants "beacon out" their fields of concerns, exploring the extent of their investigation through dialogue, then focusing on salient features to be recorded. They suggest the following basic procedures:

- Leave a 10-second gap at the beginning of each tape
- Make a trial recording to ensure equipment is working
- Give people time to "warm up" before recording
- Check the material immediately after recording
- Stick to a designated time limit
- Allow time for people to comment after recording

Videos, however, do not reveal "the facts" or "the truth." They still provide only partial information since only small segments of time may be recorded, and the lens focuses only on particular features of the context or events, according to the particular interest or interpreting eye of the photographer. A useful way of using this particular tool is to record events identified by preliminary analyses of interview data. The camera then focuses on features of the scene identified as significant by participants in the process.

Artifacts: Documents, Records, Materials, and Equipment

In traditional anthropological investigations, understanding a cultural context sometimes required an intensive study of artifacts related to the daily social life of the setting. This is true to some extent in action research, though the focus on artifacts is somewhat different in nature. Voluminous information related to health service delivery can be found in documents and records, and useful insight may be gained by investigating associated books, materials, and equipment. A survey of the physical facilities—furniture, buildings, clinics, wards, offices, and so on—may also be instructive.

Researchers, however, need to be selective and focused since huge and unwieldy piles of information, much of which has little relevance to the issue investigated, may overwhelm an investigation. In action research, participant accounts provide a frame of reference to focus further observation. Preliminary analysis of interview data reveals the features and elements of experience or context that might benefit from the gathering of additional information. Comments like "I hate the diagnostic machine were using. It's so frightening," or "These new instruments are the best thing since sliced bread," may lead to a review of machinery and equipment used in the clinic.

Participant perspectives as revealed in interviews, therefore, provide the central point of reference for reviewing artifacts. Ultimately, however, material is collected according to whether or not it appears pertinent to the issue investigated. Whether medications, furniture, clinic facilities, or other items are included becomes evident when they are included in participant interview responses. Reviewing interview field notes or transcripts, therefore, enables researchers to identify artifacts to be included in the study.

Documents

Researchers can obtain a great deal of significant information by reviewing documents in the research context. Patient files and records, organizational procedural manuals, and duty statements may provide crucial information about factors involved in the delivery of health care within the setting. At the clinic or ward level, policy documents may include rules and regulations providing insight into institutionally approved behaviors, activities, or procedures. Policy documents can also provide information about the broader health system. These may be complemented by annual reports containing details of the structure, purposes, operations, and resources of the health service organization. Memos, meeting minutes, procedure statements, departmental plans, evaluation reports, press accounts, public relations materials, information statements, and newsletters likewise extend out understanding about a health organization and its operation.

In some environments, documentation is prolific. Researchers need to be selective, briefly scanning a range of documents to ascertain the information contained and its relevance to the project's focus. They should keep records of documents reviewed, noting any significant information and its source. In some cases, researchers may be able to obtain photocopies of relevant documents.

In reviewing documents and records, research participants should always keep in mind that they are not finding "the facts" or "the truth." Information is always influenced by the authors or written in accordance with particular people's motives, agendas, and perspectives. This is as true at the organizational level as it is at the level of the individual, since people or groups in positions of influence and power are able to inscribe their perspective, values, and biases into official documents and records. Documents and records, therefore, should always be viewed as just information from another source or stakeholder, having no more legitimacy or truth value than any other stakeholder.

Records

Confidential records often are not available for public scrutiny, and researchers may need special circumstances and appropriate formal approval to gain access to them. Where research is "in-house," however, review of records can often provide invaluable information. Individual files detailing client histories, case notes, charts, and district or state records may provide information central to the investigation (see

Treatment plans	Research reports
Intervention protocols	Demographics
Training programs	Statistics
Case reports	Databases
Client histories	
Client charts	Legislation
	Rules and regulations
Posters	Policies and procedures
Manuals	Annual reports
Research papers	Budgets
Reference lists	Archives
Bibliographies	
Medication manuals	Constitutions
	Meeting minutes and agendas
Work portfolios	Rosters
Performance appraisals	Correspondence
Attendance records	Emails
Case records	Memos
	Reports
Diaries	
Calendars	Circulars
Phone logs	Notice boards
Car logs	Pamphlets and brochures
Schedules	Educational materials
Appointment books	
Mileage records	

Figure 4.4
Documents and Records

Figure 4.4). Comparisons with similar health service organizations may reveal interesting information, providing much needed perspective to an investigation. Perceptions that a health service organization is poorly funded, or that a particular client group has low access to services, may not be borne out by a review of the records. As with all information, however, such information needs to be carefully evaluated since much of it is recorded in statistical form requiring careful interpretation. In circumstances where statistical information is used, the research team needs to include someone with the relevant expertise to interpret the information acquired.

Client Case Notes

Client case notes provide a wonderful resource for investigation, providing highly informative information. They enable research participants to review a chronological record of the types of activity in which health professionals and clients engage. Information from case notes provides a useful addition to other data, but should be collected parsimoniously, since they tend to accumulate with astonishing speed.

As with other artifacts, case notes should be selected according to their relevance to the research issue, and therefore should be gathered after preliminary analysis of interview data has provided the means to focus selection of this information.

Materials, Equipment, and Facilities

A review of material and equipment provides useful input to the investigation, since there is a vast array of artifacts that are involved in health service delivery. From hospitals to small neighborhood clinics, health services contain a large variety of instruments, machines, and equipment that are employed in client care. A range of medications and associated storage devices, ventilators, home dialysis equipment, blood sugar machines, blood pressure machines, and special aids for the disabled and frail-aged are also found in client homes. All of these artifacts of health care are housed in buildings that are constructed and organized in particular configurations affecting and determining the way services are delivered.

Research participants should carefully review materials, equipment, and facilities as part of their observations (see Figure 4.5). As with other observations, the focus and direction of reviews will be determined by information acquired in interviews. Researchers should be wary of focusing on details that participants interpret as having little significance to the issue investigated.

Newspapers	
Journal articles	Medications
Magazines	Medication aids
Television reports and documentaries	
Radio	BP machines
Films	BSL machines
Photos	Weighing machines
Maps	Ventilators
Posters	Drip stands
	Catheters
Rooms	Shunts
Space arrangements	Hoists
Lighting	X-ray machines
Ventilation	Anaesthesia equipment
Air conditioning	
Heating	Furniture
Storage facilities	Computers
	Televisions
	Projectors

Figure 4.5
Materials, Equipment, and Facilities

A health service where I visited was located in an old warehouse in the inner city. The downstairs waiting room and clinic and consulting rooms had no windows to the outside world. Services for aged-care clients were provided in a building across the street, and the health promotion unit that provided community outreach services was located in yet another building further down the block. Unsurprisingly, the physical layout of the building had extremely negative effects on staff communication and client access.

Recording Information

As researchers review artifacts, they should take careful note of information they consider relevant to the investigation. They should list information they have reviewed, together with a summary description of the nature of the material. In the process, they should record which information may be made public and which must be kept confidential. The intent of the summaries is to provide stakeholders with information about materials that might enhance their investigation. If, for instance, stakeholders have a perception that a client's health status is declining, then access to appropriate records will enable them to check whether or not this is so. This information will enable participants to extend, clarify, or enhance existing issues and perspectives as they emerge.

Surveys

A survey is another means of providing input into an action research process. Unlike "quasi-experiments" that use statistical analysis to test a hypothesis, surveys are sometimes used in action research to acquire information from larger groups of participants. A survey may be used, for instance, to acquire information from a particular client group. The major advantage of surveys is that they provide a comparatively inexpensive means to acquire information from a large number of people within a limited time frame. Their disadvantage is that it is frequently difficult to obtain responses from those surveyed, and the fixed nature of the information that can be obtained by this means. Surveys are best conducted in the latter stages of an action research process when stakeholding participants have had opportunities to frame the research issues in their own terms.

Creswell (2002) describes the different ways surveys can be administered—self-administered questionnaires, telephone interviews, face-to-face interviews, computer-assisted interviews, and website and internet surveys. He suggests that there are two basic survey designs: a cross-sectional design that collects information from people at one point in time, and a longitudinal design studying changes in a group or population over time. Surveys always obtain information about people's perspectives on an issue, rather than their actual behaviors. A study of client perspectives on services provided by a clinic, for instance, may focus on client attitudes, beliefs, and opinions, or elicit information about their perceptions, feelings, priorities, concerns, and experiences of a particular service. The latter is more appropriate for action research, which focuses largely on revealing the perspective and experience of participants.

Researchers may increase the validity of a survey by ensuring that it is grounded in concepts and ideas that more closely fit the experience and perspectives of those surveyed, by doing face-to-face interviews with a small sample of participants (see "Interviewing: Guided Conversations," page 60). They may then use that information to formulate questions for the survey instrument. Surveys can be conducted through face-to-face interviews or through paper and pen questionnaires, and each may be administered to individuals or groups. Paper and pen questionnaires are useful when researchers require specific information about a limited number of items, or when sensitive issues are explored.

Questions in action research surveys may be comparatively unstructured and open-ended to maximize opportunities for respondents to answer questions in their own terms, or highly structured to acquire specific information related to issues of concern.

Conducting a Survey

- **Determine the purpose, focus, and participants.** Prior to constructing the survey instrument (questionnaire), carefully define:
  - Issues to be included
  - The type of information to be obtained
  - The people from whom it will be acquired

- **Formulate questions.** Ensure that questions:
  - Cover all issues and all types of information identified
  - Are clear and unambiguous
  - Do not include two issues in the one question (e.g., Are clinic hours adequate and at the right times?)
  - Are framed in positive terms, rather than negative
  - Do not contain jargon likely to be unfamiliar to respondents
  - Are short and to the point

- **Responses.** Provide appropriate response formats. Formats should provide sufficient space for responses to open-ended or semi-structured questions. Closed response questions may take the following forms:
  - **Open response:** e.g., How many minutes should be allocated for a consultation? _____minutes
  - **Fixed response:** e.g., How frequently should the community health nurse visit—daily_____, every two days_____, every three days_____, weekly_____, other_____.
  - **Dual response:** Responses choosing between two alternatives—e.g., yes/no, agree/disagree, male/female

- **Rating response:** e.g., Using the following scale, circle the most correct response 1 (strongly disagree), 2 (disagree), 3 (neutral), 4 (agree), 5 (strongly disagree)

- **Provide framing information.** Inform potential respondents of the purpose and nature of the survey. Include information about the likely duration of the interview/session, and the types of response required (e.g., extended responses or precise responses).
- **Trial.** Test the adequacy of the questions by having preliminary interviews or questionnaire-completing sessions with a small number of people. Modify questions that prove to be inappropriate or ambiguous.
- **Administer** the questionnaire or conduct the survey.
- **Thank** people for their participation.
- **Analyze** the data.

Where more complex, extended, and/or analytic surveys are contemplated, researchers should use appropriate sources to ensure effective valid designs (e.g., Bell, 1993; Cook & Campbell, 1979; Creswell, 2002; Fink, 1995; Oppenheim, 1966; Youngman, 1982).

Statistical and Numerical Data

Health services generate large amounts of numerical data related to client well-being, including diagnostic data, progressive charts of the client's vital signs, case notes with dosages, and test results indicating the levels of a multitude of indicators, as well as data concerning organizational inputs and outputs, inventories, and financial statements. Other sources of quantitative data that may enhance an action research process include information included in official reports and records, as well as that available in epidemiological studies and research reports.

Unlike experimental research, where statistical data is used to test hypotheses, action research uses numerical and statistical data as another form of information to extend or clarify participant understandings of an issue or problem. Surveys also provide numerical information that can be used to test the applicability of specific concepts and ideas to broader populations. Numerical and statistical data are particularly useful where there is a lack of clarity about the occurrence of particular phenomena. Depending on the nature of the study, statistical information may provide descriptive information related to:

- **Occurrences** of a phenomenon (e.g., the number of clients who attend a clinic, the number of patients suffering a particular illness)
- **Comparisons** of different occurrences (e.g., comparisons of clients with different illnesses, differences in the occurrence of a condition in men and women)
- **Trends, or history** of occurrences over time (e.g., whether the number of smokers in a population or sample is decreasing over time)
- **Central tendencies** (e.g., measures of the mean blood sugar readings of a particular client, or group of clients)

- **Distribution of scores** (e.g., whether there is a wide spread of body-mass index readings among clients, or whether most have similar readings)
- **Correlations** that measure the degree of relationship between any two phenomena (e.g., whether hours of exposure to sunlight correlates with the occurrence of skin cancer amongst a client group)

Inferential or analytic statistics are often used in epidemiological studies. Such techniques as analysis of variance, multiple regression analysis, factor analysis, and so on, assist researchers to determine the effect of different factors on a phenomenon of interest (e.g., the extent to which the prevalence of a particular disease may be attributed to or affected by exposure to sunlight, toxic chemicals, or genetic inheritance). A wide range of epidemiological studies has been amassed in the research literature, providing a rich body of information with the potential to inform research participants about particular health issues.

Rarely, however, does statistical data provide "the answer" to an issue or problem, since the information must first be interpreted to understand precisely what it is saying and to judge its relevance to the people and the setting of any study. Part of the job of qualitative interpretation, therefore, is to find out what the numbers are saying, to ensure that people understand the significance of the information, to clarify what it means in terms of the issue investigated, and to assess its relevance to the current context. It is important, however, that people ensure that "all the evidence is in," since it is easy to extract the results of a single study, or to focus on one part of a table of statistics and interpret them out of context. As with all other information, quantitative data needs to be carefully interpreted to ensure that it assists in clarifying and extending understanding emerging in the study.

Reviewing the Literature

Reviewing literature is an ongoing facet of stakeholder processes of inquiry. As issues and perspectives emerge, the literature review becomes more focused, enriching the information base of the investigation. In action research, the literature is positioned quite differently from that in traditional academic research, being viewed as the source of other views or perspectives rather than as the source of truths or facts. Facts, according to Frus (1994), are social constructions, as much in need of investigation and exploration as other features of the context. Literature reviews also should be quite thorough to ensure that limited perspectives are not used as ammunition to force particular types of action.

In an action research process, therefore, the literature might best be seen as another set of perspectives, providing useful information to be incorporated into the perspectives and accounts emerging in the research process. In Figure 4.6, nurse and client perspectives are obtained through interviews, analysis of which provides understanding of stakeholder experiences and perspectives on an issue. A review of literature may reveal perspectives, interpretations, or analyses emerg-

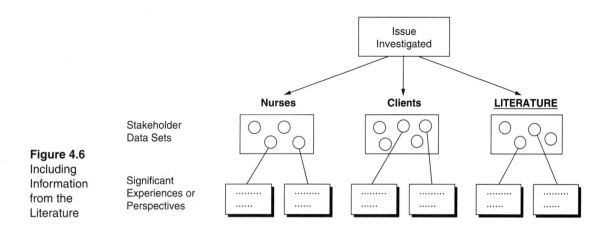

Figure 4.6
Including
Information
from the
Literature

ing from other studies of that issue, or provide discrete information related to a particular condition or treatment—providing research participants with information that can enhance, complement, or challenge the constructions emerging within their study.

Processes for Reviewing/Deconstructing the Literature

A variety of sources may contain useful literature that speaks to the issue investigated, including academic texts and journals, professional journals and publications, and institutional or departmental publications and reports. These may include accounts of successful practices, projects, or learning processes, demographic information pertinent to the location or group studied, or indications of factors likely to have an impact on the study. They also may provide information about previous research on the issue, existing programs and services, or accounts of similar projects. Care needs to be taken in applying generalized information to the specific site of the study, however, since it is possible that the conditions in the setting, or the nature of particular groups, differs significantly than those from which other studies are drawn. Although they may provide generalized analyses of an issue, the results of other studies may not provide the basis for action in any particular local setting.

The literature is not a body of truth, however, since studies may be comprised of a range of different theories, diverse ways of conceptualizing an issue, and different assumptions, values, and ideologies embedded in the research texts. These often unrecognized assumptions and sets of ideas sometimes are either inappropriate to the research in which participants are engaged, or unconsciously impose a way of conceptualizing a situation or an issue that fails to take into account the concrete realities facing people in their specific situations. Part of the researcher's task, therefore, is to deconstruct the literature, revealing the inherent concepts, ideas, theories, values, and ideological assumptions embedded in the texts of their writing.[1]

Reviewing and deconstructing the literature requires participants to:

- Identify sources containing information relevant to their investigation
- Distill the main features of lengthy articles or reports
- Identify information, concepts, or ideas that illuminate or resolve emerging issues
- Deconstruct concepts and ideas, revealing unintended preconceptions, assumptions, or biases
- Include distilled information in ongoing processes of reflection and analysis

A review of the literature may incorporate materials in libraries, community organizations, government agencies, or on websites. Often, material may be accessed through computerized search processes and databases. Research participants may use a web search engine to locate resources or gain assistance from the help desk at their local or university library. They should be wary of using abstracts, however, since they often contain distorted or poorly formulated information. If a piece of literature seems pertinent, then it should be read in full text form.

Using the Literature Review

As information from the literature enters the research cycle, participants can make decisions about its worth or relevance. It may provide information enhancing or confirming the perspectives already reported, or challenging the views and experience of stakeholder participants. The literature may also contain information suggesting actions to be taken or provide examples of actions taken in similar contexts. For formal reporting procedures, an extended review of the literature also provides evidence that participants have thoroughly investigated a variety of sources of information and taken this into account in their investigations.

Information emerging from the literature review, therefore, may be used:

- As part of the ongoing processes of reflection and analysis
- As information to be included in emergent understandings
- As material to be included in reports

---

[1] The emphasis on deconstruction is another facet of qualitative research. Quantitative research assumes value-free or value-neutral research generalizable to all contexts. Qualitative research highlights the cultural and context-specific nature of knowledge, and the importance of understanding an author's perspective, since they often infer truths about an issue on the basis of their own experience and perspective and fail to take into account the often different experiences and perspectives of those about whom they write.

Developing Insight: Emergent Understandings

As participants accumulate information from a variety of sources they acquire the materials from which new understandings emerge that enable them to gain greater insight into people's experiences and perspective. This provides a substantial body of information that will enable them to take action to remediate the issue or problem that provided the focus of the study. The information may be encapsulated in reports detailing the outcomes of the research (Chapter 6, page 118), or in practice frameworks providing the basis for changed practices (Chapter 7).

As indicated in Figure 4.7, participant accounts derived from interviews provide the primary material for constructing emerging understandings, incorporating as they do information that resonates with the experience and perceptions of research participants. These preliminary accounts, however, are modified, clarified, enriched, or enhanced by information from other sources. Information from observation, together with material derived from reviewing documents, records, and other artifacts, may extend and enrich accounts derived from participant perceptions. Insightful or useful information may also be obtained from the literature reviewed during the processes of inquiry.

The accounts and understandings emerging from these processes of data gathering and analysis are not static, however, and continue to be enriched, enhanced, and clarified as researchers enter continuing cycles of the process, adding further information from the same or other sources. The continuing Look-Think-Act cycle may incorporate information from the diverse sources identified in previous sections of this chapter.

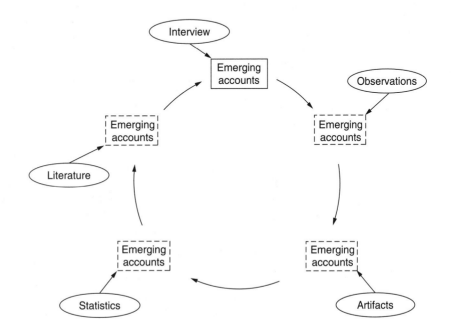

Figure 4.7
Building the Picture:
Emerging Accounts

Figure 4.7 typifies the process of data collection, though the reality is messier, since information and analysis converge in the research arena from a variety of sources, sometimes serendipitously, and at odd moments in the research process. The art and craft of research is in the skilful management of this diverse body of information, distilling and organizing data into a coherent and clear framework of concepts and ideas that people can use for practical purposes.

SUMMARY

Gathering Data: Sources of Information

The major purpose of this part of the research process is to gather information from a variety of sources. *Stakeholder experiences and perspectives* are complemented by *observations* and reviews of *artifacts and literature*.

This process requires research facilitators and other participants to develop *trusting relationships* enabling the easy interchange of information.

The *interview* is the primary tool of data gathering, providing extended opportunities for stakeholders to reflect on their experience. Key features of the interview process include:

- ***Initiating* interviews**
- ***Grand tour* questions to elicit participant responses**
- ***Mini-tour* and *prompt* questions to extend participant responses**
- **Using *focus groups* to work collaboratively**

Information is also acquired through *observing* settings and events.

A review of *artifacts* provides a rich additional source of information. These may include:

- **Records**
- **Documents**
- **Work samples**
- **Materials, equipment, and facilities**

***Numeral and statistical information* from these sources, or from a survey, can provide other useful resources.**

Academic, professional, and institutional *literature* also provides useful information to extend participant understandings.

***Accounts and reports* will emerge developmentally as information accumulates through cycles of investigation.**

Giving Voice:
Interpretive and
Qualitative Data
Analysis

5

RESEARCH DESIGN	DATA GATHERING	DATA ANALYSIS	COMMUNICATION	ACTION
INITIATING A STUDY	CAPTURING STAKEHOLDER EXPERIENCES AND PERSPECTIVES	IDENTIFYING KEY FEATURES OF EXPERIENCE	WRITING REPORTS	CREATING SOLUTIONS
Setting the stage			Reports Ethnographies Biographies	Care plans
Focusing and framing	Interviewing	Analyzing epiphanies and illuminative experiences	PRESENTATIONS AND PERFORMANCES	Case management
Literature review	Observing			Problem-solving
Stakeholders	Reviewing artifacts	Categorizing and coding	Presentations Drama Poetry	Enhancing practices
Data sources	Reviewing literature	Enhancing analysis	Song Dance Art	Evaluation
Ethics			Video Multimedia	Health promotion
Validity		Constructing category frameworks		Community development
				Professional development
				Strategic planning

Contents of This Chapter

This chapter presents detailed procedures for two approaches to data analysis.

It commences by explaining the *purpose* of data analysis in naturalistic inquiry/qualitative research.

The first data analysis section presents procedures for analyzing *epiphanies or illuminative experiences*. The main thrust of this method is to identify and *deconstruct*, or "unpack," epiphanies (significant experiences) to reveal the key features of participant experiences.

The next section describes *categorizing and coding* procedures for analyzing data. Researchers *"unitize" the data*, and identify discrete pieces of information people reveal in interviews, then select and sort data into a *system of categories*.

Introduction

The following framework signals the move from data gathering to data analysis. In terms of the simple Look-Think-Act of action research, the Think component indicates the need for participants to reflect on the information they have gathered to transform the sometimes large and unwieldy body of information into a relatively compact system of ideas and concepts that can be applied to solutions to the problem at hand (see Figure 5.1).

The purpose of data analysis is to sift through the accumulated data to identify the information that is most pertinent to the issue on which the study has focused. This process of distillation provides the material for an organized set of concepts and ideas that enable stakeholders to achieve greater insight, understanding, or clarity about events of interest. One of the essential features of action research is the move to ensure that this process captures directly the experience and perspective of all participants to ensure that it makes sense to them all.

This differs from common research practice, in which data analysis is driven by categories and schema derived from a particular theoretical perspective. In such situations, theoretical formulations often dominate proceedings, inscribing academic perspectives into the process and silencing the voices and perspectives of other participants. Though there is still a need for objective research that engages these types of practice, action research focuses more clearly on a phenomenological approach to analysis that starts with the "local" theories of the research participants.

This chapter first presents an approach to data analysis that seeks to preserve participant perspectives by using "epiphanic moments" (Denzin, 1989b)—illuminative or significant experiences—as primary units of analysis. The ultimate intent is to give voice to those participants, revealing key meanings in their language and providing a body of ideas and concepts that clearly mesh with important elements of

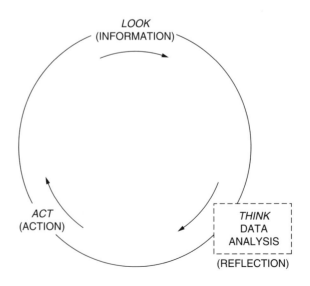

Figure 5.1
Reflection in Action Research

their experience. The second process presented is a more traditional form of qualitative analysis—categorizing and coding data that distills large amounts of data into a more manageable body of ideas. The purpose of this process is to formulate a system of concepts that reveal patterns and themes within the data that expose the key features of events and settings.

Tight schedules and multiple commitments make it difficult for health professionals to stand back and reflect on their work. When they have the luxury of an opportunity to sit back, talk about, and reflect on the their health service or management practices, they often gain significant insights into their professional life. I've frequently seen a health professional's eyes light up in the course of interviews or focus group dialogues as they see themselves or aspects of their work in new ways. Merely having time to focus their attention in a systematic way is illuminative.

This does not always happen immediately, however. The realization that persistent confrontation with abusive relationships was an experience that permeated and affected much of their practice came slowly for a group of community health workers with whom I worked. As they built trust in each other and shared their stories, they gained deep insights into their practice (Genat, 2001). The process of analyzing their experience enabled participants to extend their understanding of issues and provided concepts and ideas that enabled them to devise effective actions related to the problems they experienced in their work. Data analysis, for them, was not just a technical research routine, but the means to inform their actions.

Data Analysis (1): Analyzing Epiphanies

The processes of inquiry described in this book largely emerged from the history of research in the academic disciplines. While action research has much in common with the general methodologies of naturalistic inquiry/qualitative research, its purposes are distinctively different. Traditionally, research has sought to provide scientific, objective theories of human conduct, providing conceptual schemes to explain how and why people act as they do. Action research, however, uses these types of theory as background information, choosing to focus instead on the ways people purposefully construct and make meaning of their social worlds. The intent is to understand the ongoing, experienced reality of people's lives rather than to seek an objective truth that explains observed events.

Data analysis reveals how people make sense of their experience and utilizes these understandings to enact positive change in their lives. The focus of interpretive research on meanings people give to themselves and their life experiences requires researchers to capture the voices, emotions, and actions of those studied in order to acquire an empathetic understanding of another's life experience. The following analytic procedures provide the means to identify those aspects of experience from which we can formulate accounts of the events, actions, activities, behavior, and deep emotions that make up the ongoing reality of human experience (Denzin, 1997). They utilize methods that enable the voices of the participants, their structures of meaning, their interpretive processes, and their conceptual frameworks to structure and guide data analysis (Genat, 2001; Young, 1999).

The procedure is based on a methodology of interpretive analysis suggested by Denzin (1989b) with a focus on *epiphanies*—illuminative moments that leave marks on people's lives. By exploring and unpacking these epiphanies and illuminative moments, we seek to reveal features and elements of experience, often not apprehended in the normal course of events, that provide significant insight into events in people's lives.

Epiphanies and Illuminative Experiences

Epiphanic experiences are illuminative moments of crisis or transformational, turning point experiences that result in significant changes to people's perceptions of their lives (Denzin, 1989).

They may vary in intensity, from the life-shattering experience of complete failure or triumphant success, to less calamitous events that have significant, but not dire, effects on people's lives. They emerge as moments of human warmth or hurt, or moments of clarity that add new dimensions to a person's life experience, investing them with new ways of interpreting or understanding their lives. An epiphany may emerge instantaneously—the "ah-ha" experience, the "light bulb" that enables a person to say "so that's what is going on"—or it may emerge gradually, through a cumulative sense of awareness that emerges over an ongoing process of experience and reflection. Rhonda Petty reveals how she came to understand the concept "epiphany". She (Petty, 1997, p. 76) writes:

> *When I first read Denzin's (1989) definition and description of epiphanies I associated them with psychotic behavior or life-threatening diseases. My interpretation was too narrow. As Denzin wrote, epiphanies are turning-point experiences, interactional moments that mark people's lives and can be tranformational. My own experience demonstrates, however, that epiphanies can stem from the unlikeliest of sources—a book, a conversation, or the click of a telephone.*

Recently, I interviewed a health service clinic client who revealed, in the course of a very ordinary discussion, the results of a blood test. As she spoke of her disappointment and fears, the tears welled up in her eyes. She described the effect those results were likely to have on her family and work life and, in the process, revealed much about her family life, her approach to her work, and her relationship with her family members and work colleagues. In this case, the real life that existed beneath the surface of her apparently ordinary life provided significant insight into her family and work experience.

Epiphanies may be positive or negative, may vary in intensity and emerge instantaneously or more gradually. They are moments of truth that change or give added meaning to people's lives and therefore provide a means to move toward descriptions and interpretations of lived experience more clearly representing the lifeworld of the people studied. When shared with others as stories or narratives, they provide key meanings central to the narrator's experience and provide significant insight into the key elements participants use to construct and give meaning to their ongoing lives.

Interpreting Epiphanies and Illuminative Experiences

Interpretive data analysis commences with researchers reviewing the research problem and identifying epiphanic or illuminative experiences related to that problem. Each epiphanic or illuminative experience is then deconstructed (or unpacked) to reveal significant or underlying features, using the terminology, concepts, and structures of meaning embedded in participant accounts. By starting with events significant from participant perspectives, we seek not only to give voice to participants, but also to reveal understandings that emerge from, resonate with, and are consistent with the world as they know and understand it. We seek emic (insider) constructions that are true to their worlds and their purposes.

We are not only interested in individual accounts, however, but wish to understand the experience of different groups. Nurses, clients, and family members, for instance, are likely to see the same issue from quite different viewpoints. We, therefore, formulate joint accounts providing insight into the perspective and experience of each stakeholding group.

Figure 5.2 shows how data related to the perspectives of nurses, clients, and family members is analyzed and used as the basis of a report on a health service issue. To accomplish an interpretive analysis, researchers will:

- Review the *issue, question, or problem* on which the research has focused.
- *Assemble and review the data*, including field notes of stakeholders' interviews and focus groups.
- *Select data* related to individual participants *(key people)* who have experiences that are either particularly significant and/or typical of members of their group, in relation to the issue investigated.
- For each of those individuals, identify *epiphanies or illuminative (significant) moments* within their experiences.
- Deconstruct, or "unpack," descriptions of those experiences to reveal the *features and elements* of which they are constructed.
- Use those features and elements to construct *individual accounts* describing how each person experiences and interprets the issue investigated.
- Review individual accounts to *identify common and divergent features* and elements of experience within each stakeholding group.

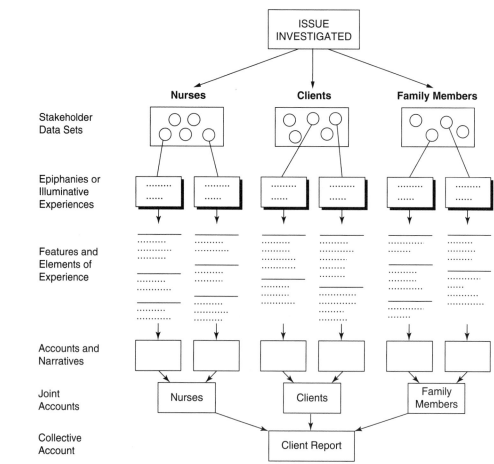

Figure 5.2
Analyzing
Epiphanies

- Use this material to construct *joint accounts* revealing the significant perspectives and experiences of each stakeholding group.
- Finally, review joint accounts to identify common and divergent features and elements of experience *across or between groups.*
- Use across-group material to construct a *collective account.* The collective account provides an overall version chronicling events by comparing and contrasting the perspectives of the different stakeholding groups within the setting. It identifies points of commonality of perspective and experience, and points of discrepancy, diversity, or conflict.

In action research, points of commonality provide the basis for concerted action, while discrepant perspectives, viewpoints, or experiences signal the need to negotiate agendas and actions around unresolved issues.

Selecting Key People

Often, it is not possible to work with all individuals in a context because of constraints of time or resources. It is sometimes necessary to focus attention on a smaller number of people to explore their experience in depth and to reveal with clarity the elements and features of experience that have a significant impact on events. The purpose of selecting key people, therefore, is to identify those individuals whose experiences or perspectives seem either typical of other people within the setting, whose experiences or perspectives appear particularly illuminating or significant (Creswell, 2002), or who are likely to have a strong influence on the emerging course of events.

Sometimes persons may be chosen because other people in their group hold them in high esteem, or because their contribution to the life and work of the group is seen as particularly significant. Significance may, however, be interpreted in negative as well as positive terms. The perspective of a client whose behavior is disruptive, or a nurse who constantly complains about clinic organization, may be as illuminative to a research process as that of a highly valued client or staff member.

Key people may be thought of as those likely to provide important information or to have a significant impact on events within the organization. In commencing interpretive analysis of data, research participants will select a number of persons from each stakeholding group, ensuring that they choose people who:

- Represent diverse perspectives from within the group
- Are likely to have a significant impact on the group
- Have seemingly typical experiences and perspectives
- Have particularly unusual or significant experiences or perspectives

Participants may be used to assist in identifying key people, as researchers ask questions like "Who do you think might provide useful perspectives on this issue?" or "Who in your group would give me a quite different perspective?"

The first step in interpretive data analysis, therefore, is to identify those people from within each stakeholding group whose combined experiences and perspectives will provide the material from which an understanding of that group will be drawn.

Identifying Epiphanic or Illuminative Experiences

The next move—identifying epiphanic or illuminative experiences—has no magical recipe for revealing the true or real epiphanies. Rather, data analysis commences with a process of selecting those events or features of a person's experience that are especially significant in relation to the issue investigated. Sometimes they are most evident when strikingly significant events emerge within the research process itself or are revealed in accounts presented in interviews. At other times, however, judgments are made on the basis of an intimate knowledge of the person, events, and the context that comes from extended engagement. Significant or epiphanic events are identified according to the expression of the participant.

The first reading of the data by a researcher, therefore, requires an empathetic, interpretive analysis responding to the internal question "What are the most significant experiences for this person (in relation to the issue investigated)?" The participant's descriptions of events provide clues, but the complex nuances of emotion and non-verbal cues displayed in interviews also provide information suggesting those events that might usefully be singled out for further analysis. Sometimes significant events or features of experience are self-evident, the participant providing animated, agitated, or emotional descriptions of events and experiences that touch their lives in dramatic and consequential ways. At other times, a more focused and subtle reading is required to identify those features of experience that have a significance impact on the lives of the persons involved. Sometimes it is evident in the extent to which the person focuses on a particular event or experience, in the person's tone of voice, their language and terminology, their countenance, their body language, or the emphases given to certain events.

> Within focus group discussions a group of health workers shared their experiences working to service a cohort of clients. As one individual shared an experience, others would reflect on their experience of similar situations and their own unique responses. As they discussed the particular kinds of situations they encountered when visiting clients in the community, one exclaimed:
>
> "I think we create dependency . . . I'm not a lawyer, and I've been spending all week at court—I'm not a lawyer—I'm a health worker—and I feel like everything that I've learned, like all the paramedical stuff—that's not important!—it's all the social stuff—I feel like the social takes over—more than the paramedical or anything to do with medical . . . like I can see the point of someone going with them [to court]—it's just that it seems it is always the health worker—and it should be the family, or even welfare agency's job . . . health workers—see this is what I mean—it's like the jack-of-all-trades . . . when you are doing all these other things . . . there's not enough of a person to go around."
>
> This outburst of frustration reveals crucial elements of this worker's experience: She feels frustrated by the multiple demands made on her; she believes that a community health worker should provide predominantly clinical or "paramedical" services rather than social services; she fears fostering dependency amongst the clients; and she feels other people should be responsible for many of her activities. Initially, these emerged as key features of one community health worker's experience. Subsequent analysis of data revealed them as important features of her colleagues' experience (Genat, 2001).

Epiphanies and significant events, therefore, take on a range of complexions, both in terms of their intensity and their meaningfulness to participants. Sometimes a relatively trivial event can create great emotion, while at other times what appear as momentous events create little response. The following examples indicate illuminative moments that signaled epiphanies emerging from data analysis:

"If he does that one more time I'll scream!"

"Is she just dumb? I've explained it to her six different ways and she just doesn't get it."

"I'm clear! I'm clear! I'm clear! I'm clear!"

"Oh, Jane. That is just wonderful. I knew you had it in you."

"It was so important that we did this work ourselves. If others had done it for us we wouldn't have learned anything!"

The deconstruction or unpacking of these moments provides the material from which to construct descriptions or narrative accounts. By analyzing the events and meanings surrounding these descriptions, we are able to construct an understanding of their significance. Epiphanic moments enable us to focus on those features and elements of experience that "make a difference" in the lives of participants.

Sometimes the meanings of the words are self-evident, but more usually it is necessary to provide information about the ways in which the words were delivered and associated information. It is not unusual for people to be led to tears as they speak of events with sometimes barely contained emotion. In the examples given, the meanings are reasonably clear, but it would be necessary for people engaged in analysis to take into account the levels of excitement, frustration, anger, voice tone, and body language in order to understand the significance of the words spoken. The **expression** of the words is at least as important as the words themselves.

Sometimes epiphanies are revealed unexpectedly. Many times as I've interviewed people I've been struck by the emotive force of their description of particular events. I was recently surprised, however, to find my eyes "leaking" as I was being interviewed about a cross-cultural training program in which I had been involved. Though I thought I was recounting events in a fairly objective way, I had not realized the extent to which they had moved me. The interviewer informed me that it was not unusual for people to be moved to tears as they described events within this program. I coined the phrase "ethnographic tears" as a way of indicating the possibility of engaging people's deeply felt experience within an interview.

Ultimately, however, the choice of ephiphanies or significant events requires direct use of member checking with the person concerned, and triangulation with the others, as it is easy to misinterpret or wrongly choose events in other people's lives. Ideally, when the data is member checked (i.e., when the research facilitator allows the participant to read or read back the information they have provided), the participant should be asked which events were most significant—a grand tour question (Spradley, 1979a) framed something like "What, in all this, is most significant for you?" This provides opportunities for the person to identify those events with the most impact on their own lives. You might further ask, "What is it that really moves, excites, or concerns you?" However, there is a need for care; participants may not have any part of their experience that is moving, exciting, or concerning, but nevertheless have features of experience that effect their lives or work. One step back from this is a procedure in which the researcher identifies significant events and checks their importance with the participants.

Although we focus on events, sometimes significance lies in people's actions and/or responses, or the impact of features of the environment—physical space, dress, and so on. Significance is revealed in the body-language, the non-verbal communication that gives us clues about the impact of events. A frown, a smile, a look of pain or anger, or forceful language suggests the need to focus on what is said:

> *"She's such a bitch—dressing like that and talking like that. I just can't stand being around her."*
> *"I won't work there much longer. The office is so small I can't even think, let alone do my work."*
> *"When I saw what that kid had accomplished, I almost cried. She was fabulous."*

As we explore people's descriptions of events, therefore, we review interview accounts to identify features and elements of the experience, and related features and elements that have an impact on the situation. The feature of experience, "The office is so small I can't even think," may lead us to explore related components of a participant's experience. Comments on the size of an office, in this instance, were related to the number and complexity of the person's work activities, and the space she felt she needed to store materials and do the work required of her. As became evident in reviewing the data, the work itself was the significant feature of the experience, even though the size of the office was the "straw that broke the camel's back" and became the immediate focus of the agitated comment. Identifying epiphanies and significant experiences, therefore, requires a researcher to search for significant events in people's lives, but also to make connections between related phenomena.

Epiphanies do not need to be associated with momentous events. Minor epiphanies occur quite regularly as people reflect on their experience, sometimes commenting on the "little light bulb that went on in my head" as they realize the significance of something they have described. These might be more appropriately called illuminative moments, because they reflect processes of understanding and clarity that sometimes emerge as people reflect on their own experience or hear other people's stories.

Deconstructing Epiphanies: Features and Elements of Experience

The next step in this process is to deconstruct the epiphanies, ascertaining those elements and features that enable an audience to understand the nature of the experience. We need to ask, "How is this event significant for the persons themselves? What features of this event would they see as significant?" We are, in effect, unpack-

In a health worker study, a powerful epiphany was identified within a one-to-one interview with a community health worker. She finds the work with a marginalized group of clients almost overwhelming:

"When I was going out in the field I found it really difficult to start with. It was just sort of getting to know the people and getting their trust. You sort of feel like you are just doing a sort of Band-Aid treatment out there. You're just going out there and doing the same things day in and day out with no improvement. Nothing is happening . . . you're going out there telling everyone to take their medication—that it's going to get better—if you do this it's going to get better—but it doesn't seem to get better . . . sometimes you feel what's the point—there doesn't seem to be any point in it . . . why am I doing it? The main hassle is the fact that it is the same problems—they don't go away." (Genat, 2001. p. 32)

Epiphany
Major Features   I found it really difficult to start with
                                            getting to know the people
                                            getting their trust
                                            doing a sort of Band-Aid treatment
                                            there doesn't seem to be any point in it

Key Elements (of "doing a sort of Band-Aid treatment")
                                            doing the same things day in and day out
                                            no improvement—nothing is happening
                                            telling everyone to take their medication
                                            [telling everyone] it's going to get better
                                            it doesn't seem to get better

Figure 5.3
Deconstructing an Epiphany

ing or interrogating the epiphany, seeking to reveal the embedded elements of experience. In doing so, we use information drawn from the data, and use the concepts, terms, and language of the people as they described events, behaviors, responses, and so on—applying the verbatim principal described previously (see Chapter 4).

Figure 5.3 provides an example of this process. The participant, reflecting on her experience, described how she "found [the work] really difficult to start with." Major features of this difficult work included "getting to know the people," "getting their trust," "doing a sort of Band-Aid treatment," and "there doesn't seem to be any point in it."

Further analysis of field notes indicates the elements of experience associated with each of these. Elements of "doing a sort of Band-Aid treatment," for instance, included "doing the same things day in and day out," "no improvement—nothing is happening," "telling everyone to take their medication," "[telling everyone] if you do this it's going to get better," and "it doesn't seem to get better."

Researchers will deconstruct each epiphany to reveal the different features of experience inherent in the event. Sometimes a single epiphany is sufficiently powerful to provide the basis for a detailed analysis of a person's experience, whereas other accounts may require ongoing analysis of a number of minor epiphanies, illuminative moments, or significant events.

As research participants work through this process of deconstruction, they may use other analytic frameworks that alert them to the types of information that might usefully be extracted from the data. A framework of concepts drawn from ethnographic observation (Spradley, 1979b) indicates the types of phenomena that might be used as epiphanies, features, or elements of experience. These include acts, activities, events, times, places, purposes, and emotions.

Another useful framework—**What, Who, How, Where, When, Why**—also may be used to assist in identifying useful or relevant detail. In all this, we are not attempting to include all possible detail—the possibilities are infinite. We do not need an extended description of the more mundane, taken-for-granted properties and features of everyday life, but we do need to identify the essential features of people's experiences or perspectives. It's important that we don't let the framework drive the data analysis process, starting with "acts" and working down through the concepts. The trigger for selecting features and elements are those aspects that are seen or felt by participants to be a central part of their experience. Framework concepts merely serve as reminders of the type of phenomena that might be included.

In all this, researchers need to focus their analysis by ensuring that the information revealed is associated with the issue or question that provides the focus for the study. They should ask, "How does this event illuminate or extend our understanding about the issue we are investigating? Does it provide answers to the questions that assisted us to frame our study?" In some cases, the analysis will reveal information indicating the need to extend the boundaries of the study or to focus on issues that were not part of the original plan. The iterative or cyclical nature of the research process enables us to build understanding and extend our study accordingly.

Epiphanies in Observations and Representations

Sometimes epiphanic moments occur in the course of observing events and activities within a research setting. Any health setting is likely, over a period of time, to experience disruptive events that disturb their relatively orderly routines and procedures. A client outburst, conflict between a health professional and client, or an altercation between staff members signals an epiphanic event that may provide worthwhile focus for further exploration. The event itself tells part of the story, but description and analysis by participants reveals the meanings and experiences associated with the event that have the potential to greatly increase understanding about the issue investigated. Significant events, therefore, provide the focus for follow-up interviews to enable participants to explore and deconstruct events and explore the meanings embedded in singular events. A single event sometimes provides more insight into the underlying structures of behavior, or the ways everyday events are experienced or interpreted by the people involved.

Constructing Conceptual Frameworks

Once epiphanies have been deconstructed, revealing the key features and elements inherent in participant experiences, the analyzed information is organized into a carefully structured system of concepts that help people to clearly understand the import of what has been revealed. This structured system of concepts not only provides a summary of important information, but also supplies the basis for writing reports and planning actions.

The following sections provide examples of how deconstructed epiphanies—the analysis of significant events within two action research projects—provided the framework for written accounts of each.

Case Example: Deconstructing an Epiphany

The following excerpt, taken from a study of community health workers, demonstrates the way unpacking a description of an epiphanic event provides the framework for a report on health worker roles.

Ruby shares her concerns about the scope of health worker practice in a defining moment. Her acute exasperation leads her to question the mandate of health workers to provide the appropriate, and indeed extraordinary, health services necessary. Following a particularly frustrating staff meeting with clinic staff, she sits with her colleague Merle at the kitchen table in the staff room. Slumped to one side, gloomily resting her cheek in her cupped hand, she broods pessimistically on the potential of health workers to change the health status of the community.

"They wanted all us health workers 'cause we were going to change everything but we're so strictly dictated to it's changed nothing — some of us have great ideas and we could do it all but we just can't do it—instead of like—handing things to us. We're always dictated to . . . we don't get enough say in the program . . . I thought yes we've got a power, we're united, but then last week it just killed it . . . we say we want to have our own voice! You should'a been there—there were all these powerful health workers that just agreed to everything [the nurse] said . . . people are still dying—Teddy's going to get his toes cut off—Daisy died . . . people are just dying of things that could have been changed; I mean they may just as well employ nurses."

Ruby's narrative reveals her anguish at the recognition that neither she nor her colleagues have sufficient authority to make a significant impact. Despite claims about the central role of Aboriginal health workers, Ruby finds that they are unable to effect any notable changes. In her view, this is because other health professionals control their work. At the same time, she perceives that her own people are needlessly suffering and dying. Not only does she observe that health workers have few opportunities to make change individually, but also that they have limited collective power. Laboring under the dictates of other professionals, Ruby suggests that health workers are unable to provide a service distinct from the service provided by community nurses. Consequently, she concludes that health workers lack any discernible professional identity. (Genat, 2001. p. 142)

This epiphanic event provided the basis for an ongoing analysis of health worker roles. The following framework of headings indicates the end result of the analysis. Situating Health Workers in the Health System

Lacking Professional Identity, Voice, and Status: "We don't get enough say"
Dominating Doctors: "We're always dictated to"
Unrecognized, Disbelieved, and Dismissed: The case of Teddy
Marginal in the Planning Process: "We have great ideas"
The Case of Daisy: "We don't get enough say"
Summary: "Health Workers were going to change everything . . . but it's changed nothing"

Using People's Terms and Concepts: The Verbatim Principle

As we engage in data analysis, it is particularly important to use the terms and concepts from the participants' own talk to label concepts and categories. The temptation to characterize people's experience in terms that seem to make more sense or clarify the issue from the researcher's perspective, or to translate it into language fitted to theoretical or professional discourses, should be clearly resisted. Later, when the need for joint accounts incorporating diverse terms, concepts, and ideas emerges, we may need terminology that allows us to collectively describe similar elements or features with one term or phrase. "I was angry," "She made me feel bad," "I nearly cried when he did that," and "I'm just scared what he'll do next," may be elements of a feature described as "The Emotional Impact of . . ." Generally, however, we should seek terms from within the speech of the participants themselves, adding additional words only to clarify meaning or extend understanding when the words themselves are insufficient for the purpose.

> Maria Hines, a member of a city neighborhood group, is most explicit about her experience of analyzing data in a project in which she participated. With a slight frown, she describes how "I never knew how difficult it was *not* to put my own words and meanings in. We had to really concentrate to make sure we used what people had actually said and not put in our own words. It was *hard*."

These words remind us to focus clearly on one of the central features of action research, consciously seeking to understand the perspective of others and to use those perspectives to formulate actions. This is centrally important at the stage of data analysis, where the possibility of reinterpreting or misinterpreting people's words, concepts, and ideas—taking them and using them for our own purposes—is ever present.

Data Analysis (2): Categorizing and Coding

Another common process of data analysis in qualitative research is based on procedures for sorting units into categories, each of which is denoted by a label—a conceptual code. The process is very useful for analyzing large bodies of qualitative data and is especially amenable to computerized data analysis. It runs the risk, however, of losing participant perspectives in conglomerating data from a wide diversity of sources, and of revealing conceptual structures meaningful mainly to those responsible for data analysis. Using participatory processes of data analysis can minimize both of these weaknesses.

Purposes and Processes of Categorizing

The purpose of analysis in action research is not to identify the facts or what is really happening, but to distill or crystallize the data in ways enabling researcher participants to interpret, understand, and make meaning out of the collected materials. Initially this involves the identification of commonalities, regularities, or patterns within in the data.[1]

The process commences by reviewing interview and focus group data, dividing them into units of meaning—unitizing the data—then using these to construct an organized system of categories and themes (see Figure 5.4). This system of categories then provides the basis for research reports and accounts and for ongoing action agendas. Continuing analysis incorporates data from observation, artifact reviews, or from literature reviews.

Reviewing the Research Question

When it is time to begin the formal analysis, research participants have two primary sources to draw from in order to focus and organize the analysis:

- The research questions generated during the planning and design phase of the project
- Analytic insights and interpretations that emerged during data collection

---

[1]Harry Wolcott (1994) suggests description, analysis, and interpretation as the three purposes of data analysis, the latter being generalized theorizing not specifically relevant to the context at hand. The type of analysis presented herein makes no distinction between analysis and interpretation, as Harry depicts them. The purposes of action research require "theorizing" or "interpretation" that makes sense from the perspective of participants. Generalized theory, more relevant to theory building in the academic disciplines, has less relevance to our current purposes, though it often assists in framing the study. Shirley Bryce Heath (1983), for instance, used ethnographic methods for studying children's language use in different communities. Both data gathering and analysis were affected by understandings about the types of things associated with or affecting children's language, resulting in descriptions of the communities of people. The "interpretive lens" filtering information was that provided by socio-linguistics.

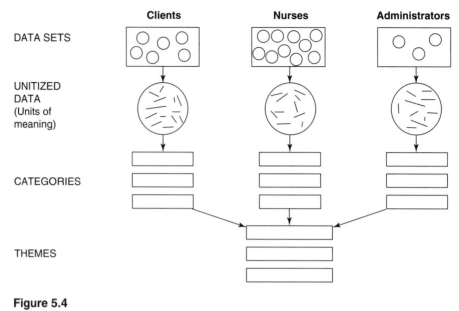

Figure 5.4
Categorizing and Coding

Reviewing the research questions ensures that participants focus their analysis in ways relevant to the purpose of the study, and maximizes the potential for outcomes that point to tangible and productive outcomes.

Reviewing Data Sets

Different groups of stakeholders often experience events in different ways. In health care settings, for instance, clients often experience and interpret events quite differently from health care providers or administrators. Male clients often have different experiences and perspectives than female clients, and nurses have quite different perspectives than doctors. Client experiences and perspectives are likewise likely to differ according to the clients' age, family background, religion, race, ethnicity, and so on.

Generally, therefore, we formulate data sets to acknowledge the important distinctions existing between stakeholders in a setting. In Figure 5.4, for instance, data from clients, nurses, and administrators is analyzed separately, revealing points of commonality and difference in their perspective.

The purpose of reviewing the data sets is to familiarize researchers with the data, enabling them to take an overall view of the information so that links between items and elements begin to emerge. Those responsible for data analysis should therefore commence by reading through all the data.

Unitizing the Data

The next step in the process is to isolate features and elements of experience and perspective to focus on the specific details emerging from people's talk about events and experiences. Data recorded in interviews and focus group sessions is first printed, and then divided into *units of meaning*. A unit of meaning might be a word, a phrase, a part, or the whole of a sentence. The sentence "I don't really like the way I organized this class because it's too one-dimensional and I prefer to work thematically" has a number of distinct units of meaning. These include "I don't like the way I organized this class," "the class is too one-dimensional," and "I prefer to work thematically." As indicated here, it is sometimes necessary to add words to a unit so it makes sense when it stands alone.

A variety of methods are used for this purpose. Some researchers isolate units of meaning by physically cutting sheets of interview data with scissors, while others use highlighters to isolate units of meaning related to emerging categories. Computer programs such as NUD*IST, Ethnograph, Nvivo, WinMAX, and Hypersearch are also used to engage in this process electronically.[2] Computer-assisted programs, however, provide only a data storage, managing, and searching tool. They cannot engage in analytic processes such as identifying units of meaning or formulating categories.

The process of unitizing the data results in a large "stack" of discrete pieces of information. From these building blocks, researchers sort, select, and organize information into an organized system of categories that enables participants to make sense of the issues they investigate. The next phase of the process of analysis, therefore, is to categorize and code units of data.

Categorizing and Coding

Spradley's (1979a) schema for *componential* analysis, similar in concept to analysis of *units* of meaning, provides a useful conceptualization of the process of categorization. Spradley's approach to analysis is based on the idea that people's everyday cultural knowledge is organized according to systems of meaning. These systems of meaning, he proposes, are organized taxonomically, using an hierarchical structure to distinguish the different types of phenomena that might be organized as categories. Categories divide and define our cultural worlds systematically, allowing us to impose a sense of order on the multiple and complex phenomena that comprise our everyday life.

A simple set of common categories is indicated in Figure 5.5. Ingestibles—substances that can be swallowed and ingested—are comprised of food, drink, and medication. Each of these is comprised of a number of different items that comprise the category. The category "food," for instance, is made up of fruit and vegetables. The category system is incomplete, but provides an illustration of the way people organize phenomenon in order assist them to define and communicate objects.

---

[2]Reviews of these programs may be found on http://www.sagepub.com

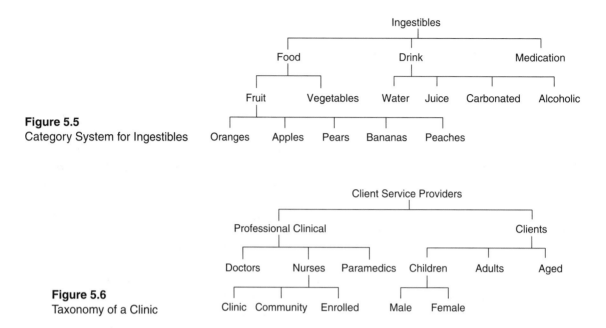

Figure 5.5
Category System for Ingestibles

Figure 5.6
Taxonomy of a Clinic

Having identified the units of meaning inherent in the interview data, researchers will then identify those associated with each other and which might be included in the same category. The example in Figure 5.6 provides a way of categorizing the different types of people involved in the delivery of clinical services.

In the taxonomy of Figure 5.6, two major types of people are identified from the data—*professional clinical staff* and *clients*. Different types of staff include *nurses*, *doctors*, and *paramedics*. Participants make important distinctions between nurses according to whether they are classified as *clinical, community*, or *enrolled* nurses. As the system of categories is organized, decisions must be made about the placement of each item into a particular category or subcategory. In the example given, there may be it need to decide whether a community nurse who has major clinical responsibilities is classified as a clinical or community nurse. Items are placed within particular categories or subcategories according to a system of inclusion, based on the attributes of each element. The categories of clinical or community nurse, for instance, are first identified by asking structural questions identifying who should be placed in each category (e.g., "Can you name all the clinical nurses here?" "Who are the community nurses?").

We extend our understanding of the reason for placing people into particular categories by asking attribute questions, which identify the reason for placing a person in a particular category (e.g, "What is a clinical nurse?"). Answers to these questions would provide the criteria employed for making a decision to define a nurse as "clinical" as opposed to "community" or "enrolled." A clinical nurse might be identified, according to the system of meanings used in this clinic, as one who:

- Works solely in the clinic
- Works mainly on curative practices

- Has no community health experience
- Is supervised by the director of clinical services
- Works alongside physicians

These attributes define a "clinical nurse" and allow researchers to make decisions about which nurses are to be included in that category.

When we place phenomena into a category, one of the principal tasks is to name that category to identify the type of phenomena it contains. Apples, pears, and oranges might be identified as fruit, for instance. This process is called coding, so that the term used to name the category is called, by some researchers, the *code* for the category.

Spradley uses the word "cover term" to refer to this term. Researchers should first determine whether an existing term occurs naturally in the language or talk of the people from whom the information has been acquired. Otherwise, they should provide a label for the category that clearly identifies the nature of the category. Fearful, mistrustful, resistant, apathetic, and compliant, for instance, might be identified by the code or cover term "client responses."

As information is placed in categories, therefore, we become aware of the need to define more clearly the meanings intended by research participants in order to understand how the word or phrase is being used, and therefore whether it should be included in one category or another. The codes or cover terms will eventually provide a structured set of categories that assist us in organizing and making meaning of the experiences of diverse stakeholding.

Categorizing and coding, therefore, requires researchers to:

- Unitize the data
- Sort units into categories
- Divide categories into subcategories, where appropriate
- Code each category using a cover term expressing the type or nature of information in the category or subcategory
- Identify the attributes defining each category or subcategory

Other formats for coding and categorizing data may be found in Bogdan and Biklen (1992), Creswell (2002), and Arhar, Holly, and Kastern (2000). These provide detailed instructions for developing descriptions and representing findings.

Organizing a Category System

As researchers formulate categories, they first place them in an organized system that clarifies the relationship between features and elements of experience. Decisions must be made about which categories are given priority and where they are placed in relation to each other. In the community health-worker project featured in Figure 5.7, major categories identified include "Paraprofessional Perspectives," "Professional Practitioner Perspectives," and "Client Perspectives," each containing subcategories revealing different elements of those perspectives. "Professional Practitioner Perspectives" includes subcategories

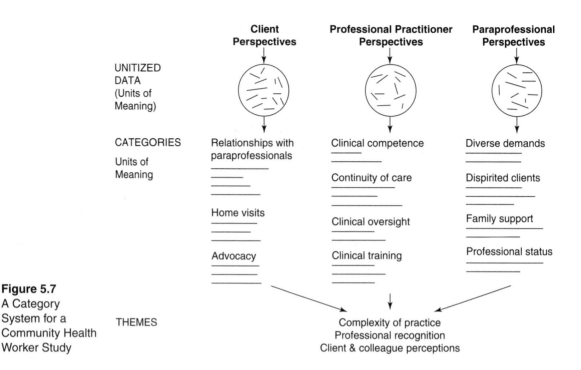

Figure 5.7
A Category
System for a
Community Health
Worker Study

"clinical competence," "continuity of care," "clinical oversight," and "clinical train-ing." Details within those subcategories are comprised of units of meaning reveal-ing people's experiences or perspectives of those issues. Note that there is no right way of organizing the data. It might as easily have been organized with "clinical competence," as a major category, and paraprofessional, professional practitioner, and client perspectives presented as subcategories. The general process is de-picted in the concept map of Figure 5.7.

In Figure 5.7, categories have emerged for Clients, Professional Practitioners, and Paraprofessionals. The first cluster of units of meaning (category) for Client Per-spectives is labeled "relationships with paraprofessionals," the next category is "home visits," and the final category emerges as "advocacy." Although category labels provide no common elements across stakeholding groups, it is clear that some issues are related, and these have been identified as *Themes*, each identified by a code. The Client category "relationships with paraprofessionals" has been associated with Para-professional category "professional status" and identified as a theme coded "profes-sional recognition." The categories "home visits," "advocacy," "diverse demands," "dispirited clients," and "family support," have been linked as a Theme having the code "complexity of practice."

Researchers, therefore, construct a system of categories and subcategories or-ganizing the emerging information in ways that make sense to the participants. They do so by using terms or codes representing or encompassing stakeholder experi-ences and perspectives.

Enhancing Analysis: Incorporating Non-Interview Data

Thus far, data analysis has proceeded by exploring information derived largely from interviews. A variety of other data also has been gathered, however, and this has the potential to enhance or clarify information or issues emerging in the first phases of data analysis. Information acquired through observation, artifact reviews (documents, records, materials, and equipment), and literature reviews might be used to complement that information inherent in the items categorized in the preliminary analysis of data. In the previous example, for instance, interview information related to "professional recognition" might be enhanced, extended, or thrown into question by data from organizational records or reports. Likewise, perceptions about "complexity of practice" might be given more credence, or be challenged by, information from client files or from comparison with reports on paraprofessional practice in other settings. Once interview data have been analyzed, therefore, researchers should review other available information, focusing especially on information pertinent to the identified issues, features, or elements.

Other data also include information emerging from the literature review. In action research, the process of investigation is driven by participant perspectives, rather than those contained in the literature on the issue. Authors within the literature, however, might be viewed as secondary stakeholders because their writings have the potential to influence the research process. In this respect, viewpoints within the literature are treated as another set of perspectives, having the same status and validity as those of other stakeholders.

Research participants may find it fruitful to review information within the professional, bureaucratic, or academic literature that might throw light on issues and elements emerging from data analysis. There is a broad range of research that challenges many of the commonly held assumptions circulating in clinic and community contexts, or reveals the uncertain nature of many of the so-called "spray on" solutions that emerge from time to time. A thorough review of the research literature on any topic often provides a unique resource assisting people to refine their analysis of the problem investigated. Pertinent information is identified and included in the process of analysis to enhance and clarify participant perspectives.

A review of the literature related to indigenous health workers supports many of the issues revealed through Genat's (2001) study of health worker experience. They share many features and elements of experience with health workers in many parts of the world. In some instances, however, the literature challenges their perceptions. It suggests other interpretations of events, or points to the differences between the experiences of health workers across settings. The literature provides a point of reference enabling a richer understanding of health worker roles to emerge.

Non-interview data is especially important when working with young children who frequently have limited ability to talk of their experience in abstract terms. There are many other ways, however, in which children make meaning of their experience and communicate with others. We should carefully observe the ways children enact their work and play activities; the ways they talk to others; their drawings; their songs, stories, and poems; their descriptions of events; and their responses to events and activities. These artifacts help us to understand how a child makes meaning of events in his/her life and to construct accounts clearly representing the child's perspective. If we can fathom ways of making learning activities meaningful from their perspective, then our teaching task becomes so much easier and more rewarding.

Reviewing information related to children's events and activities provides richly rewarding information assisting researchers, and the children themselves, to make sense of the issue at hand. Analysis of these types of data requires interactive processes that first identify significant features or elements of experience, then check the ways children make meaning or interpret those features of experience. Researchers should review data related to:

- Observations of children's activities, or their participation in events
- Oral or visual recordings of their activities, including verbal interactions
- Drawings and artwork
- Letters
- Stories, verbal and written
- Play
- Drama

Researchers should work with children to identify significant features and elements of these types of information, constructing understandings on the basis of the way the children interpret the information reviewed.

Non-interview data, therefore, provide a variety of rich resources having the potential to enhance and clarify understandings emerging in the processes of investigation. The process is described schematically in Figure 5.8, though the cyclical nature of action research will mean that the revised analysis may be subject to further exploration using participant interviews or focus groups.

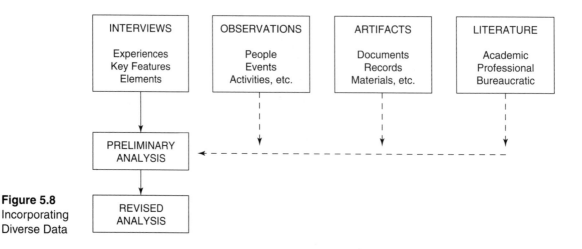

Figure 5.8
Incorporating
Diverse Data

Using Category Systems: Frameworks for Reports and Accounts

Systems of categories emerging from data analysis provide frameworks of concepts that provide a structure for reports. The Community Health Worker study, for instance, used themes and categories presented in Figure 5.7 on page 108 as the basis for framing a report:

- Introduction
- The CHW Practice Domain: Complexity of Practice
    Diverse Demands, Multiple Dilemmas: "A Jack of all Trades"
    Engaging a Dispirited Response: "You feel what's the point"
    A Breakdown in Family Caring: "They don't care"
- Client and Colleague Perceptions
    Client Perceptions of Services: "Talking to your own people"
    Doctors' Perceptions: "They don't understand clinical indicators"
    Co-Worker Perceptions: "CHWs could do more"
    Perceptions of Nurses: A Clinical Perspective on Status
- Situating CHWs in the Health System: Professional Recognition
    Lacking Professional Identity, Voice, and Status
    Interaction, Participation, and Status
    Claiming a Professional Domain

Details within the report derive from the units of meaning included within each category or subcategory. Thus, the report described previously includes a heading "CHW Practice Domain" and a sub-heading "Diverse Demands" that commences with the following text: "There's a lot of welfare stuff—and I reckon we deal more with the social welfare stuff than actually going out doing blood pressures and sugar levels and medication and that sort of thing—in my experience. I think we do a lot of welfare stuff—things like getting housing, getting food for the families." The text continues to present details of how paraprofessionals are experiencing and interpreting the diverse demands of their clients, including the full range of elements drawn from the unitized data within the "diverse demands" category.

Analyzing Data Collaboratively

Data gathering and analysis in action research is much more effective when it is accomplished as an interactive process between stakeholders. Participants share accounts emerging from individual interviews, formulate joint accounts, then return to the interview phase to reflect on and extend their own accounts. There may be a number of iterations of this process during an extended study of a complex issue (see Figure 5.9).

A similar process is envisaged in Figure 5.10, where initial focus group exploration provides a framework of concepts and themes that are used for further exploration of people's experience and perspectives. Again, the process is designed to help achieve deeper understanding and greater clarity, providing the basis for actions to resolve the issue explored.

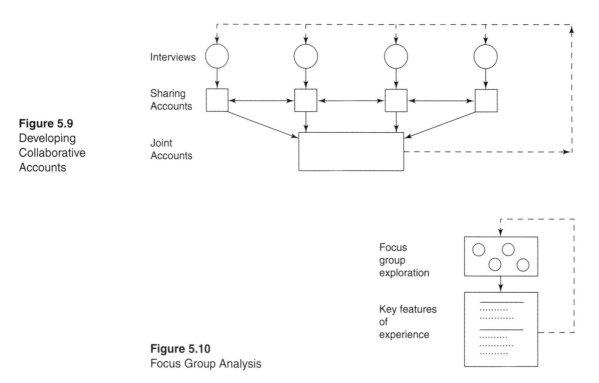

Figure 5.9
Developing
Collaborative
Accounts

Figure 5.10
Focus Group Analysis

This not only extends understanding between the diverse individuals and groups, but also enables them corporately to construct a framework of ideas for on-going collaborative action.

Over the years, I have been impressed by the amount of energy and goodwill emerging from well-prepared focus groups. Positive and productive outcomes are never certain, since a history of antagonisms or the presence of authoritarian figures may inhibit group discussions or interaction. I have experienced, however, a high degree of success in this type of activity. A recent half-day workshop with faculty within a university illustrates the types of outcomes possible. Faculty explored the use of technology in their teaching, sharing ways they currently used computers to enhance student learning and identifying future uses. The level of animation in their discussions and the extensive lists of useful information emerging from their discussions were testament to their enthusiasm and the extent to which they appreciated opportunities to learn from each other. It also provided clear direction for the project team who had set up the workshop, indicating directions to take in resourcing faculty to extend their use of technology to enhance student learning.

> The productive buzz that continued through this workshop was not the result of idle gossip or general conversation. As I walked around the room listening to group conversations to monitor the progress of their discussion, I was taken by the intensity of their focus. Group discussions focused clearly on issues of interest or concern provide a wonderful context for reaffirming the broader contexts of their professional work and reminding them of the underlying nature of the work they do together.

Conclusion

Data analysis is the process of distilling large quantities of information and revealing the central features of the issue investigated. The process of crystallizing information into a category system provides the basis for increased understanding of the complex events and interactions comprising everyday events in clinics, hospitals, homes, and community settings. Its major purpose is to provide the basis for richly evocative accounts and reports providing stakeholders with the information and understanding upon which to make informed decisions about policies, programs, and practices for which they are responsible. It also provides the building blocks for therapeutic action within the research process, clearly delineating issues and agendas requiring attention.

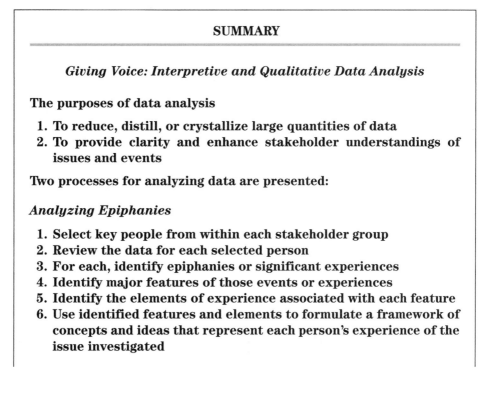

SUMMARY

Giving Voice: Interpretive and Qualitative Data Analysis

The purposes of data analysis

1. **To reduce, distill, or crystallize large quantities of data**
2. **To provide clarity and enhance stakeholder understandings of issues and events**

Two processes for analyzing data are presented:

Analyzing Epiphanies

1. **Select key people from within each stakeholder group**
2. **Review the data for each selected person**
3. **For each, identify epiphanies or significant experiences**
4. **Identify major features of those events or experiences**
5. **Identify the elements of experience associated with each feature**
6. **Use identified features and elements to formulate a framework of concepts and ideas that represent each person's experience of the issue investigated**

7. **Make connections:** Identify similarities and differences between features or elements in stakeholder experiences
8. **Use frameworks to construct accounts and/or reports**

Categorizing and Coding

1. **Review the interview data for each stakeholding group**
2. **Unitize the data: Divide into units of meaning**
3. **Formulate categories, subcategories, and themes identifying patterns, connections, commonalities, or regularities within the data**
4. **Organize these into a category system**
5. **Incorporate information from non-interview data**
6. **Use the category system to provide a framework for accounts and reports**

Collaborative Data Analysis

Focus groups may be used to analyze data and share information collaboratively.

Representation: Communicating Research Processes and Outcomes

RESEARCH DESIGN	DATA GATHERING	DATA ANALYSIS	REPRESENTATION	ACTION
INITIATING A STUDY	CAPTURING STAKEHOLDER EXPERIENCES AND PERSPECTIVES	IDENTIFYING KEY FEATURES OF EXPERIENCE	WRITING REPORTS	CREATING SOLUTIONS
Setting the stage			Reports Ethnographies Biographies	Care plans
Focusing and framing	Interviewing	Analyzing epiphanies and illuminative experiences	PRESENTATIONS AND PERFORMANCES	Case management
Literature review	Observing			Problem-solving
Stakeholders	Reviewing artifacts	Categorizing and coding	Presentations Drama Poetry	Enhancing practices
Data sources	Reviewing literature	Enhancing analysis	Song Dance Art	Evaluation
Ethics		Constructing category frameworks	Video Multimedia	Health promotion
Validity				Community development
				Professional development
				Strategic planning

Contents of This Chapter

As participants engage in research processes, they need to inform each other of their progress. At the conclusion of a project, the outcomes of research also need to be communicated to stakeholding audiences.

This chapter provides an understanding of:

- The *purposes* for reporting research processes and results
- The different means used to *communicate* this information, including written reports, presentations, and performance
- Procedures for developing *written reports*
- Procedures for preparing and staging *presentations*
- Procedures for preparing and producing *performances*

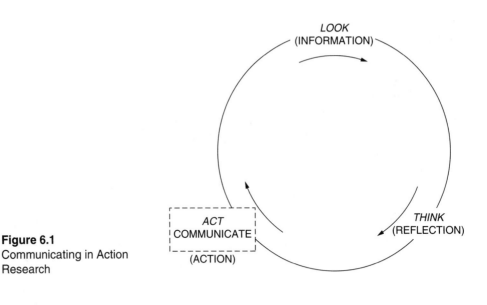

Figure 6.1
Communicating in Action
Research

Introduction

Within the Look-Think-Act framework of action research, the first Act is to present the outcomes of analysis to research participants and other stakeholding audiences (Figure 6.1). The purpose of this process is to ensure that all acquire a body of shared meanings from which to work toward resolution of the research issue. Participants need to *present* the information in a form that increases clarity and understanding for all participants and stakeholders.

This chapter presents a variety of reporting techniques that might be used to inform audiences about research outcomes, including written reports, ethnographic or biographic accounts, presentations or performances.

Communication in Action Research

Reporting research activity enables participants to review their progress systematically and resolve disputes where people have different opinions about past events and planned activities. Reporting procedures also provide the means for stakeholding groups to share their experiences and perspectives, thus providing the means by which larger audiences can extend their understanding or gain a better picture of what's going on.

Purposeful communication provides the means for all parties—health professionals, managers, clients, and carers—to understand the forces effecting the issue investigated. As participants become increasingly aware of the influences at work, they can take them into consideration and work toward mutually meaningful solutions to the problems they experience.

Research participants may, therefore, report to each other for the following purposes:

- To inform stakeholders of the processes and outcomes of investigation
- To enable stakeholders to understand each others' perspectives and experiences
- To check the accuracy and appropriateness of the information emerging from the investigation
- To provide an ongoing record of the project

(Bill)

I recently worked with a group of health professionals where the issue of communication became paramount. The group was attempting to inaugurate an association for professionals dispersed throughout the state. Their project involved an inquiry into the type of organization and internal processes that would work best for their professional group. Initially, a number of problems emerged that appeared to result from a breakdown in communication between the steering committee and their potential associates. The health professionals on the steering committee became aware of the need to inform their associates of a variety of activities pertinent to the development of the association. What became evident was that the usual forms of communication—sending notices of meetings, minutes of meetings, letters of explanation, and so on—were not wholly effective. New processes of sharing information became a priority. The steering group members found new ways of communicating with each other and their potential associates, making use of a variety of media, including electronic bulletin boards, electronic mail, and photographs, text, and video clips of meetings posted on websites. These events emphasized the problems that arise when people require messages in a format that is accessible and appropriate to the context. Many of the problems and complaints evident in early stages of the project disappeared as more effective methods of communication were developed.

Different Strokes for Different Folks: Forms of Communication

Because action research requires all participants to understand what is happening to enable them to contribute to the effective resolution of the issue investigated, information must be shared with the relevant stakeholders. The objective formal reports so common in institutions sometimes are inadequate vehicles for these purposes, being framed in formalized or technical language that is not always understood by lay audiences.

The type of report format, therefore, needs to clearly differentiate between the research audiences and purposes, as they may be pertinent to three major audiences—academic, public, and professional/organizational:

- **Academic:** University research focuses principally on the development of a *body of knowledge* shared with a community of scholars. The outcomes of research are reported in journals and books stored in university library collections. The knowledge is also passed on to students in order to *inform and educate future professionals.*
- **Public:** Research sometimes is used to *inform and educate the public* about *significant issues.* Research projects sponsored by government bodies, public interest groups, or community groups report their findings in the media, often incorporating their work into television documentaries, or sometimes presenting it as drama, either on stage or as street theatre. Thus, the outcomes of research on health risk factors and preventive health measures—such as those related to nutrition and diet or exercise and lifestyle and so on—are increasingly released directly into the public domain.
- **Professional/Organizational:** Research is increasingly used for direct *professional and organizational* purposes *to improve or strengthen programs, services, and practices.* Research outcomes can be applied directly to the development of new programs and services, or used to formulate solutions to significant problems in institutions, organizations, and community contexts. Health professionals use information acquired from research studies to better inform their clinical practices or to seek more effective solutions to health problems.

The different audiences and purposes of action research require researchers to think clearly about the reporting format that will enable them to communicate most effectively with the particular audiences with which they wish to communicate. Examples of a range of different report formats are provided in Chapter 8. These do not cover, however, the full range of possibilities, as will become evident in the latter sections of this chapter. Depending on the stakeholders, the purpose, and the context, reporting may take the form of *written reports, presentations, or performances.*

Written Reports and Accounts: Writing People's Lives

Key features and elements identified in the data analysis phase of research provide the basis for written reports presenting the perspectives of participating individuals and groups. They may be presented as:

- Individual reports
- Group reports
- Progress reports
- Evaluation reports
- Final reports

As Denzin (1997) suggests, often we are not seeking definitive or objective accounts, but evocative accounts that lead the reader to an empathetic understanding of the people's lived experience. Accounts or narratives provide insight into people's lives, recording the complex emotional world lying beneath the surface of seemingly innocuous events. This breaks into view in those special moments of triumph, success, love, struggle, loss, or discord that are often revealed as participants explore their life experiences.

In action research, therefore, we seek to produce evocative accounts, conveying accurate insights into the impact of events on people's lives. Writing evocative accounts entails more than the bland reporting of events. It requires report writers to find the textual means to evoke deeper forms of understanding. A government report that referred to the "inadequate sewage" in a community failed to evoke an understanding of the stench of excreta and the parents' ongoing fear for their children's health. Objective reports are sometimes dangerously uninformative.

Extended ethnographic accounts comprised of full, richly textured narrative provide the possibility of in-depth insight into the community and/or institutional contexts in which events are played out, revealing the interactional and emotional features of people's experience. Shorter reports such as meeting minutes, team reports, progress reports, and so on, provide more condensed accounts, but are significantly enriched if they capture the essence of people's experience.

Life Stories: Biographies, Autobiographies, and Ethnographies

Written narrative accounts have the capacity to illuminate the often complex and deeply problematic nature of people's lived experience. In contrast to psychological case studies that interpret individual behavior from within a framework of disciplinary theory (personality, behaviorism, etc.), biographies and ethnographies provide the means to understand people's lives from their own perspective; to describe their lives from their own points of view.

Often the mere act of telling their own story is therapeutic, revealing to the individuals concerned features of their lives they had inadvertently repressed, or that they had taken-for-granted as a necessary though damaging feature of their lives. Conversely, it may reveal hidden positive dimensions of experience, enabling them to see their worlds in a more positive light or to come to awareness of potentials they had not been aware they had.

I have witnessed many situations where people have been greatly enlivened by opportunities to tell their stories and listen to the stories of others. In client homes, staff meetings, workshops, program development projects, and many other arenas I have experienced the joy that comes from this process. What I see is not only a sense of worth emerging from people who feel, sometimes for the first time in their lives, that someone is really listening to them; that they have something worthwhile to share with others. I am no longer surprised, but always feel gratified, when people express their appreciation in the most heart-felt terms. On more than one occasion, people have burst out in the moment or quietly informed me later "This changed my life!"

Something quite wonderful happens in the process. Not only does the storyteller experience the exuberance of being heard and acknowledged, but in the process they learn something significant about themselves and their professional or personal experiences. It is illuminating and sometimes revelationary. I have often seen people—storytellers and/or audience—in tears as their stories emerge. The teller does not need to be a practiced orator. Sometimes the straight recounting of events by simply spoken people—moms, old folk, children—has a dramatic impact on an audience; the presence of the people themselves speaking volumes. When people tell stories of their lives, it is no small thing.

The process of writing personal accounts of experience as part of an action research project is not intended to reveal the facts or the truth of a person's life, but to enable them to look at their lives in different ways; to reinterpret events, experiences, and responses; and to come to new ways of understanding their situation. Autobiographical and ethnographic accounts provide potential useful resources, enabling individuals and groups to reevaluate their place and their interaction with others in the context; to ". . . connect and join biographically meaningful experiences to society-at-hand and to the larger culture- and meaning-making institutions . . . " (Denzin, 1989a, p. 25).

Ethnographic accounts largely have been written by external authors, but we now recognize the potential for individuals and groups to write autoethnographies, self-referential processes of exploration presenting accounts of their own lives.

Joint and Collective Accounts: Connecting Stakeholder Experiences

While individual stakeholder stories reveal singular experiences relating only to one person, they often share significant experiences or perspectives with other stakeholders. Further, although they may not share the same experience, participants may be affected by the same events in different ways. We need to make connections between stakeholder experiences, therefore, in order to develop an understanding of the dynamic interactions between individuals and groups. When individual stakeholder epiphanies and features of experience have been identified, therefore, we search for connections with others. To develop joint accounts, research participants will:

- Focus on each epiphany or significant experience for each individual
- Review the data related to each epiphany

- Identify features and elements of experience for each epiphany
- Identify commonalities among stakeholder experiences or perspectives
- Record differences in experience and perspective

By comparing information within groups and across groups, we are able to make judgments about the extent that experiences or perspectives of events are commonly held within a group or shared with other groups. We are thus able to identify those singularly important experiences and perspectives that need to be taken into account in formulating solutions to the problem investigated. The terminology used in reports reflects the extent of commonality—"All clients in this study. . . ," "Many clients shared a concern about . . . ," or "While some clients indicated . . . others were more inclined to . . ."

Joint accounts (Figure 6.2), therefore, provide a summary of individual accounts, but focus particularly on commonalities and differences revealed through cross-analysis of key elements of experience. Common or similar features, in this case, may be thought of as themes.

Collective accounts present an overview of the experience and perspective of each of the major groups, so that a case report may comprise features and elements drawn from each of the stakeholding groups—nurses, clients, and physicians (see Figure 6.3). Commonalities revealed in these accounts provide the basis for collective action, while points of difference suggest issues requiring negotiation (see Guba & Lincoln, 1989), so that appropriate steps can be taken to defuse or resolve potential conflicts.

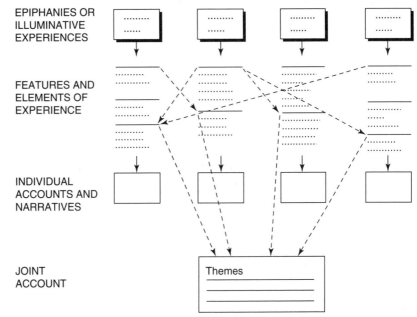

Figure 6.2
Formulating Joint Accounts

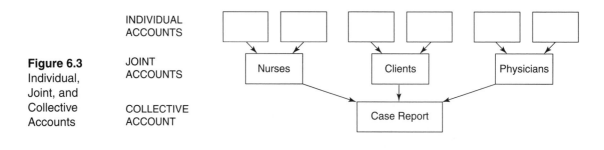

Figure 6.3
Individual,
Joint, and
Collective
Accounts

In a recent research project, analysis of data revealed that many physicians and community health workers expressed similar ideas about a communication breakdown between them. Although each perceived the same problem, they sometimes expressed it from their different sides of the coin—for instance, physicians felt that community health workers should attend clinic consultations in order to translate and articulate the needs of the frail-aged clients without recognizing that the community health workers had a full case load and commitments to clients in the home. The community health workers suggested that they were "on call" to physicians who looked down upon them, had little respect for their expertise, and rarely acted on their advice.

Sharing of this analysis provided the basis for changes to the recording and filing of the records of home visits to frail-aged clients, making them more effective for both physicians and community health workers. Whereas previously the administrative and organizational structures hindered communication between the two groups of professionals, their input into the creation of new systems produced a solution that worked for all stakeholders.

Accumulating Knowledge and Experience

Though systematic documentation takes time and energy and requires support from administrators, in the long term, accumulated notes, reflections, and reports in themselves comprise an invaluable resource that significantly supplements a practitioner's professional capacities. Professionals not only gain knowledge and skills that greatly enhance their work practices, but also acquire information that informs and enlivens their day-to-day work with clients.

Written reports may, therefore, provide a historical record of significant events and projects that add to the vitality of the culture of the clinic and the community. At the clinic level, documentation provides the means for client perspectives to be incorporated into records. A written record of specific events and projects may create a stronger sense of togetherness between colleagues and clients and assist the formation of a healthy community. Research reports, therefore, have the capacity not only to assist in developing solutions to particular problems, but also to contribute to the culture of clinic and community.

Constructing Reports

Constructing effective and useful reports is an art form in itself and becomes increasingly effective as people become more practiced. By following some fundamental processes, however, most people can write an informative report containing relevant information and conveying emerging understandings. Those responsible for writing a report should:

- Define the *audience and purpose* of the report
- *Identify participants*
- Identify the significant *features and elements of experience*
- Construct a *report framework*
- *Write the report*
- *Review and edit* the report
- *Member check*

Audience and Purpose

Carefully define the audience and purpose of the report. Ask:

- For which particular people (or type of people) will this report be written? For clients, health professionals, administrators, family members, client carers, or other significant stakeholders? In which locations—a particular clinic, a specific section of a health service organization, a nursing team on a ward in a hospital, or clients in their homes?
- For what purposes will the report be used? To inform people of progress on a project, assist them to understand features of people's experience, or reveal required actions?

Participant Perspectives

Decide which participant perspectives—individuals or stakeholding groups—are to be included. Note:

- Whose experiences or agendas are central to the report?
- Which people have important or significant associated experiences or agendas?
- Isolate the data for each of these individuals or groups

Review the Data

- Read the data relevant to the identified participants to become familiar with the material
- Note particularly evocative quotations illustrating key features of people's experience
- Note the terminology and language used by participants to describe their experience

Identify Significant Features and Elements of Experience
- Review the analyzed data to identify relevant material for the report
- Copy the key features and elements of experience for each individual or group

Construct Report Framework
Use the features and elements of experience to construct a framework for the report (see Figures 5.2, 5.7). Note:

- Key features as headings or subheadings
- Elements or units of meaning as the content of each heading/subheading

Write the Report
Write the report using the framework as a guide, incorporating the terminology and language of participants in the body of the narrative. The framework guides the writing process, but is not by itself sufficient to adequately capture people's lived experience. Reports need to encompass the multiple dimensions of human experience, including emotional, physical, and interactional elements of behavior and perspective, as well as organizational and procedural components.

The framework guiding data collection is useful as a checklist for what can be included in a narrative—people, acts, activities, events, purposes, emotions, places, times, and objects. In all this, it is important for the words of participants to provide the vocabulary and language of the report. Not only should they provide the wording of headings in the report/account, but unitized data may be strung together to form major sections of the account. Quotations may also be used prolifically to clearly illustrate the points made or the contexts described.

In a study of allied health workers undertaking community outreach work, a common theme within their experience was to feel like "A Jack-of-all-Trades." This experience was incorporated into the section heading of a chapter on allied health worker practice as Diverse Demands, Multiple Dilemmas: "A Jack-of-all-Trades," along with related subheadings in the vernacular of allied health workers. These emerged from the narratives. For instance, one worker observed, "I feel like everything that I've learned, like all the paramedical stuff—that's *not* important!—it's all the *social* stuff. I feel like the social takes over—more than the *paramedical* or anything to do with medical."

The heading Diverse Demands, Multiple Dilemmas: "A Jack-of-all-Trades" incorporated the following subheadings drawn from the speaker's words:

A Holistic Approach: "The 'social' takes over the 'paramedical'"
Vulnerable to Co-Option: "Colleagues don't see our case load as important"
Discriminating Dependency: "She wants my life"
Constantly Reconciling Dilemmas: "Not enough of you"

The report should include:

- An introduction revealing the purpose and general contents of the report
- A brief description of the context, drawn from interview and observational data
- Accounts encompassing the key features of stakeholder experiences and perspectives
- Quotations capturing significant features or elements of experience
- A concluding summary highlighting the major features revealed in the report and the implications for action relevant to the issue investigated

Review and Edit

Review the report and check that:

- Its stated purposes have been accomplished: Does the report provide adequate and appropriate information to inform the intended audience?
- All relevant participant perspectives have been included
- The language is appropriate for the intended audience
- The report accurately reflects the perspectives and experiences of participants, rather than that of the author or one stakeholding group

> (*Ernie*)
> Whenever I'm facilitating report writing, I continually ask the author the question, "Who is speaking here? Whose perspective is being presented?" Within action research, we need to use evocative language to capture the voices and experiences of the key stakeholders and to ensure we are true to their issues and agendas. It is surprising how often even the most careful report writer will allow his own perspective to intrude. When we write accounts, we must take great care to ensure we don't unwittingly present material reflecting our own perceptions and interpretations of the situation. The exceptions are those situations where we overtly include our perspective as a participating stakeholder in a research process.

Member Check

Give a draft to those about whom the report is written:

- Provide time for them to read and respond
- Talk with them in person, if possible, or by phone if not
- Check for accuracy, sufficiency, and appropriateness of information contained in the report
- Modify or correct according to their input

Report Formats

Reports will vary widely in style, detail, and length, according to the purpose of the report and the intended audience. Progress reports to research participants may be no more than a short summary of the key points emerging from prior stages of the research. In other cases, extended reports provide detailed information for the benefit of administration or funding authorities. Formal reports for funding, professional, or academic bodies—annual reports, evaluation reports, theses, or dissertations—often require a meticulous rendering of the research process in highly structured ways.

Reports will vary in format according to their function as:

- Case management reports
- Care plans
- Meeting minutes
- Informal progress reports
- Memoranda reporting on current activities and issues
- Formal reports for administrative and professional audiences
- Academic reports for publication in research journals
- Theses and dissertations

Presentations: Creative Communication

Presentations provide exciting ways to communicate research results to participants and stakeholding audiences. Constructed from multiple materials and using diverse presentational modes, they can captivate audiences by powerfully presenting participant perspectives and illuminating key features of the research. Though direct verbal addresses from prepared papers are still common, many presentations involve creative and innovative approaches incorporating charts, overheads, or electronic materials or roundtable interactive presentations, poster sessions, and structured dialogues.

Such flexible formats are especially relevant in contexts where lengthy written reports may actually inhibit communication with important stakeholding audiences. Some adults and children, especially those from poorer or culturally different contexts, may not have sufficient familiarity with professional or technical language to enable them to read lengthy formal reports. Further, written reports are often an inadequate vehicle for expressing the full range of participant experiences. They fail to convey the emotional, interactional features of experience, the nature of their social circumstances, or the complexities of their cultural realities.

Presentations, where carefully prepared and authentically presented, provide the means for more clearly and effectively communicating the concrete reality of people's lives and the elements that need to be taken into careful account when taking action. As with written reports, presentations need to be carefully and creatively planned to suit the audience, the purposes to be achieved, and the outcomes expected.

Audiences and Purposes

Research participants need to identify carefully their audience and purpose. The major questions to be asked are "What information should be presented?" and "How can we communicate most effectively with this particular audience?" In health service contexts, audiences of nurses and physicians may require different types of presentations than clients and family members.

Presentations, therefore, will vary according to purposes to be achieved. Short, informal presentations will assist participants in communicating the progress of activities to monitor the progress of their work. More detailed and carefully structured presentations may be necessary to inform a key stakeholding group—administrators, funding body representatives, supporters—of issues emerging from their inquiries to garner support for their actions.

The type of presentations will also be affected by desired outcomes. If participants wish to generate a clear or deeper understanding of people's experience, then they will prepare presentations designed to achieve that effect. Multidimensional, evocative presentations will provide a clear picture of significant events, the context in which they occur, and their impact—rational, physical, emotional, and spiritual—on the lives of participant stakeholders. This is a more emotive presentation seeking to engender understanding of the dynamics and complexities of people's experiences and perspectives. Where an audience needs to focus on more practical issues for planning purposes, then the presentation may take a more didactic form, focusing on key features and elements of the issue investigated.

An action research study on drug use among youth in a rural town identified a wide range of groups who had a substantial stake in the project. These included parents, teachers, policemen, health clinic staff, city council workers, and welfare agency staff. Each of these audiences demanded particular kinds of information in particular formats. The parents who had little experience of solvent use by young people responded to verbal presentations of stories from other parents who already had experience responding to the problem. Teachers responded to written reports outlining strategies to keep students and the environment safe. Written reports were supplemented by presentations by experts that provided knowledge of interventions that had worked elsewhere. Clinic staff were presented with written resource materials that outlined emergency intervention protocols and information about agencies to which clients could be referred. Police and welfare agency staff engaged productively in joint information sessions with parents and youth who were keen to both share their troubles and collaborate in creative problem solving. City council members and the funding body obtained written reports that assisted them in planning drug-related services and activities.

Planning Presentations

Well-planned presentations ensure that stakeholding audiences are well-informed, which enables them to maintain clarity and gain deep insights into the issues investigated. Research participants will use similar processes to report writing for planning presentations, defining:

- Audiences   Who are the audiences to whom we wish to present?
- Purposes   What are our purposes in presenting to this audience?
- Understandings   What do we want our audiences to know or understand?
- Content   What information or material will assist in achieving this purpose?
- Format   What presentational formats might best achieve this purpose?
- Outcomes   What do we wish to achieve, and what outcomes are desired?

Steps in Planning

- Identify the audience and purpose
- Identify participants whose experiences and perspectives are pertinent to the presentation
- Review the data for each of these participants
- Review the categories and issues emerging from analysis of data for each participant
- Use categories to construct a framework of headings
- Write a script, using units of meaning and/or elements within the data
- Review and edit the script, checking for accurate rendering of participant perspectives and appropriateness to audience
- Member check by having participants read the script
- Practice the presentation

The basic outcome of presentation planning is an outline or script presenting the information in easily accessible form. An outline in bulleted form provides a script that guides people's presentations. The script may be complemented by additional material, including quotations from people's talk or documented information to be read verbatim to an audience. For more formal presentations, people may rehearse their presentation to ensure they are clear about the material to be presented and to keep their presentation within the allotted time.

Research participants, therefore, need to carefully prepare a script that has the following basic format:

Introduction

The focus of the project—the issue investigated
The participants
The purpose and desired outcomes of the presentation

Body of the Presentation

Previous and current activities: What has happened, is happening
Key issues emerging from research: What has been discovered; what is problematic
Implications: What needs to be done (actions, next steps)

Conclusion
Review of major points covered

Presentations should be carefully scripted and directed so that each participant knows precisely where and when to speak, and they know the material for which they are responsible. Practice provides both clarity and confidence, maximizing the possibility of an informative and effective presentation. This is especially important for people who are not used to speaking publicly, their inclusion—the effect of people speaking for themselves in their own voice—dramatically increasing the power of a presentation.

In rare situations should people read from a pre-prepared written report. Though these types of presentations provide people with feelings of safety and accuracy, they usually detract from the purpose of the event. The written word is different in form and function from the spoken word, and people reading from a paper usually fail to convey the meaningfulness that is a necessary function of a presentation. We have all experienced presentations, delivered in mournful monotone or excited exuberance, that rattle or drone on and on. Usually, there is far too much information for the audience to absorb and little opportunity to process that information. Rarely do audiences in these situations gain appreciable understanding, and retention of information is limited. Presenting an address by reading from a pre-prepared paper is an art that few possess.

Members of a neighborhood collective planned a presentation to a national conference, a rather grand event that seemed somewhat imposing to them. After carefully identifying the purpose of their presentation—the major message they wished to present to a largely academic audience—they carefully reviewed the material they had accumulated, identifying and assessing those features that appeared central to research in which they had engaged. These features were ordered into a framework of ideas—headings and subheadings—and persons allocated to take responsibility for the various sections. They rehearsed their presentation a number of times, re-allocating some material to different people or places until each participant was clear on what they needed to say and when.

The actual presentation at the conference was highly successful, providing the audience with a clear understanding of the power of community participation in a research process. The degree of engagement of the audience was evidenced by their rapt attention and the diversity of questions they asked. The participants were highly delighted by the success of their presentation, an event that further heightened their research skills and feelings of empowerment.

Enhancing Verbal Presentations: Audio-Visuals

Though parsimonious verbal presentations can sometimes be effective, it requires a skilled and practiced orator to hold an audience for an extended period. Interest and understanding is greatly extended when visual and auditory materials are incorporated into presentations, aiding in clarity and enabling significant quantities of factual information to be presented.

A variety of visual aids complement and enhance verbal information. Diagrams, maps, concept maps, symbolic representations, figures, and so on, provide effective ways for presenting information and focusing attention. Whiteboards or chalkboards also enable the active construction of illustrations and diagrams to stimulate attention and enable the structured exposition of a wide range of subject matter. Statistical summaries, numerical information, or lists of features and elements may be presented in chart form or as overheads. Charts have the advantage of providing a constantly available record of issues, but suffer sometimes from problems of size. Overheads and other electronic means of displaying information have great clarity, but can only be projected one frame at a time, placing significant limits on the flexibility of a presentation.

Presentations can also be enhanced by electronic media in the form of audio or video recording or electronic presentations derived from such software as Power-Point. It is important to ensure that these are used in moderation, since extended use of videos or electronic media can be detrimental to a presentation, creating a passive audience and detracting from feelings of engagement. Judicious use of electronic media, however, can provide vivid illustrations or large bodies of information, greatly enhancing people's ability or willingness to participate in ongoing dialogue. As a stimulus, they are sometimes unparalleled.

At each stage, therefore, we need to ask how we can best achieve the types of understanding we desire. Presentations can be greatly enhanced by using:

- Maps
- Charts
- Artwork
- Concept maps
- Lists
- Figures
- Overheads
- Audio recording
- Video recording
- Electronic presentations

(*Ernie*)

For some years, colleagues and I have provided workshops on cultural sensitivity or race relations for a variety of audiences. The intent was to help them investigate ways of modifying their professional work practices to ensure greater effectiveness in cross-cultural contexts. These sessions have been greatly enhanced by having participants view short segments of a video film showing indigenous people presenting accounts of their experiences. One popular segment presents an old man talking of the time police and welfare officers came to take away his children. Moved to tears, he narrates the way he was prevented from taking any action as his children were driven away. Returning the next day, he describes how he put a piece of old tin over the only remaining reminder of his children, their footprints in the sand. This

> segment, used many times in workshops and presentations, never fails to evoke rich and sometimes intense discussions. It provides keen insight into the way past events continue to affect community life. Sometimes a picture *is* worth a thousand words.

For some audiences, presentations may take on an almost concert-like appearance. Creative presentations may incorporate a variety of materials and performances (see the following sections) providing a rich body of factual information and authentic understandings of people's lived realities. Presenters may incorporate tape recorded information derived from participant interviews and read from reviewed materials, or they may incorporate segments of video or oral recordings, poems, songs, or role plays. The rich variety of possibilities enables audiences of children, youth, and adult participants to fully express the ideas with which they have been working.

Interactive Presentations

It is difficult to stimulate interest or involvement in a research process when the audience is passive and uninvolved. At regular intervals, audiences should have opportunities to participate in the unfolding presentation by commenting on issues, asking for clarification, or offering their perspectives on issues presented. As part of an "hermeneutic dialectic"—meaning-making dialogue—these processes not only enable people to extend and clarify their understanding, but also increase their feelings of inclusion and ownership in the project at hand.

Presentations may also include small group work, enabling participants to explore issues in greater depth or peruse related documents or materials. Feedback from small group discussions provides a further means to gain greater clarity and understanding, especially about points of contention or uncertainty. It is possible for presentations to take the form of a workshop or focus group so that audiences become active participants in the ongoing development of the presentation.

> *(Ernie)*
> When I work with research groups, I often have them chart the key elements of their recent activities. Each group then speaks to their chart, reporting on their progress and any issues arising. The audience is able to comment or ask questions to clarify or extend the presenter's comments. This not only informs the audience clearly, but assists the presenters in extending their thinking about the issues raised—an integral part of the process of researching.

Performances: Representing Experience Artistically and Dramatically

Performances extend the possibilities for providing deeper and more effective understandings of the nature of people's experiences. They present multiple possibilities for entering people's subjective worlds to provide audiences with empathetic understandings that greatly increase the power of the research process. Performances enable participants to report on their research through:

- Drama
- Role play
- Song
- Poetry
- Dance
- Visual art
- Electronic media

The use of artistic and dramatic media permits researchers to capture and represent the deeply complex, dynamic, interactive, and emotional qualities of everyday life. They can engage in richly evocative presentations comprehensible to children, families, cultural minorities, the poor, and other previously excluded audiences.

Poetry, music, drama, and art provide the means for creating illuminative, transformative experiences for presenter and audience alike, stimulating awareness of the different voices and multiple discourses occurring in any given social space (Denzin, 1997; Prattis, 1985). They provide the means to interrogate people's everyday realities by juxtaposing them within the telling, acting, or singing of stories; thus revealing the differences that occur therein and providing the possibility of therapeutic action (Denzin, 1997; Trinh, 1991). While performances fail to provide the certainty required of experimental research, or to reinforce the authority of an official voice (Atkinson, 1992), they present the possibility of producing compassionate understandings promoting effective change and progress (Rorty, 1989).

This is clearly a postmodern response—performances make possible the construction of evocative accounts revealing people's concrete, human experience. Performances allow participants to:

- Study the world from the perspective of research participants
- Capture their lived experience
- Discover truths about themselves and others
- Recognize multiple interpretations of events and phenomena
- Embed experience in local cultural contexts
- Record the deeply felt emotion—love, pride, dignity, honor, hate, envy—and the agonies, tragedies, triumphs, and peaks of human experience embedded in people's actions, activities, and behavior
- Connect with the audience at the level of the heart and through all the senses
- Represent people's experience symbolically, visually, or orally in order to achieve clarity and understanding

(Bill)

   In recent years, I have been privy to some stunning performances that have greatly extended my understanding of people's illness experience. I have seen consumer presentations that include poetry, song, role play, and art, which both moved me and evoked far-reaching insights into the contextual realities of people's illness experience. Insights from such presentations have enabled me to extend my thinking about the ways services are organized and operate. I have seen the powerful artistic work of the frail-aged and elderly provide wonderfully illuminative representations of their particular situation. I have also seen performances by health-service providers who shared their despair at their inability to extend necessary care to their clients in the face of organizational constraints. In all these, I have been surprised by the depth and extent of my responses to these performative presentations, feeling deeply "touched" by what I have seen and heard, and I have been more sensitive to the situation of the performers, their experience, and how particular issues affect their lives.

Planning Performances: Developing a Script

Performances are built from the outcomes of data analysis, using similar techniques to those used to fashion reports and presentations. Key features and elements provide the material from which a performance is produced, participants working creatively to develop effective means for representing their experience. These may be constructed as poems, songs, or drama, or represented as symbolic or visual art. As with written and other forms of representation, performances need to be conducted with a clear understanding of the **purpose** they wish to achieve with a specific **audience.** Participants should ask: "What do we wish this audience to know or understand? And how might we best achieve that knowledge or understanding through our performances?"

- Identify the audience and purpose
- Identify participants whose experiences and perspectives are to be represented
- Review the data for each of these participants
- Review the categories and issues emerging from analysis of data for each participant
- Use categories to construct a framework of key features of experience and perspective
- Write a script, using units of meaning and/or elements within the data
- Review and edit the script, checking for accurate rendering of participant perspectives and appropriateness to audience
- Member check by having participants read the script
- Rehearse the performance

Producing Performances

As with any script, there will be decisions to be made about who will perform which roles, how the setting will be designed, what clothing or costumes will be worn, and who will direct the staging of the performance (i.e., take responsibility for overall enactment of the performance).

Rehearsals are an important feature of performances, enabling participants to review the quality and appropriateness of their production and providing opportunities to clarify or modify the script. People will also become familiar with their roles, sometimes memorizing the parts they need to play, though readings may be used effectively where people have minimal time for preparation or rehearsal.

Sometimes action research requires research participants to formulate on-the-spot performances, so that role-plays requiring minimal preparation provide an effective means for people to communicate their messages. For this mode of performance, participants should formulate an outline of a script from the material emerging from their analysis, ad-libbing the words as they enact the scene they wish to represent. Role plays are especially powerful when participants act out their own parts, speaking in their own words and revealing, in the process, clear understandings of their own experiences and perspectives.

Video and Electronic Media

Although live performances provide effective ways to communicate the outcomes of research, video and other electronic media offer powerful and flexible tools for reaching more extended audiences. Not only do video productions provide possibilities for more sophisticated performances, but they enable the inclusion of people whose personal make-up inhibits them from participating in live performances. The technology now available enables video productions to be presented on larger screens, to be shown on computer screens, or to be incorporated into more complex on-line productions.

Dirk Schouten and Rob Watling (1997) provide a useful model for integrating video into education, training, and community development projects. Their process includes:

- Making a recording scheme
- Recording the material
- Making an inventory of the material
- Deciding what functions the material will serve in the text
- Making a rough structure for the text
- Making an edit scheme on the basis of the rough structure
- Editing the text

Although producing a quality video requires high levels of expertise and careful production, current technology enables even amateurs to produce short and effective products. By recording events in clinic, service, and community, practitioners and client groups can provide engaging and potentially informative productions that extend the potential of their work. This type of recording enables people to provide sometimes dramatic renderings of their experience, and to engage in forms of research from which they were previously excluded.

Video taping also provides research participants with a variety of means for storing and presenting their material. Possibilities today include storing material in videotape form, on CD/DVD disks, or within computers, and these viewed or transmitted through a variety of media, including video and DVD players, streaming video, and community television. These formats provide the possibility of reaching a wide variety of audiences or using video productions for many effective educational purposes.

Examples of Performances

Case One: HIV Awareness

A health promotion group wished to provide information about HIV in their community. They wrote a fictional script that captured the experience of a family whose son is diagnosed as HIV positive. It incorporated dramatic dialogue about sexual behaviors that had resulted in the son acquiring HIV, steps that he might have taken to reduce the risk, followed him through the experience of contracting AIDS, working through a medication regimen, and finally dying of the disease. Produced as a play and presented by amateur theater groups in towns and cities in the region, the performance provided a graphic means for educating the broader community about HIV.

Case Two: Domestic Violence

Concerned about the levels of treatment provided by her clinic to victims of domestic violence, the director of a local health clinic acquired funds for some of her staff to produce a local video about the issue. Incorporating the perspectives of victims, former perpetrators, family members, and clinic staff, it traced the history of domestic violence in some of the families and the steps that could be taken by people suffering from domestic violence. It provided a highly useful tool to inform people in the community of the levels of domestic violence in their community, and included steps that individuals could take to deal with situations they confronted in their personal lives. The video used material from recorded interviews and role plays and reenactments of events as the source material for their video.

Case Three: Community Health-Needs Survey

A nurse facilitated a community health-needs survey in a rural community. She realized that the formal report, written for the state health authority, would not be read by people in the town. She worked with people who had been involved in the survey to consider how they might effectively inform the community. Using the key elements of the report, they wove the information into a variety of forms, eventually presenting a concert that featured short verbal presentations of central information, as well as poems, songs, artwork, and short plays to communicate central features of the report.

Case Four: Alcohol Carousel and Children's School Drawings as Part of a Community Education Strategy (Allamani, Ammannati, Forni, Sani, & Centurioni, 2000)

As part of a Community Alcohol Action Research Project, 5,500 alcohol carousels were distributed during 1996 in the project's areas, where they were freely available. Samples of a consumer's association and school parents were surveyed using a questionnaire. Local key people were also interviewed using qualitative methods. In all circumstances the carousel proved to be understandable, useful, and able to elicit discussions about alcohol issues. A two-year training program in communication skills and alcohol prevention for 13 teachers in local preschools, elementary schools, and middle schools followed the research. Teachers then planned and implemented a health education program on alcohol and food issues. One outcome was nine drawings produced by the school children. The drawings were exhibited in some schools and supermarkets and were hung in city buses.

Case Five: Frail-Aged Accommodation Project

Within an inquiry into needs for the aged inhabitants of a small rural community, the health professionals, local residents, and client representatives presented the results of their investigations to a community forum. They used role plays to present common experiences of both health professionals and clients as they attempted to secure aged-care services in the district. A common theme was the somewhat superficial understanding of city health planners about the local situation. The role play dialogue incorporated references to well-known local identities and places and was laced with local colloquialisms. The inherent humor produced much laughter from the audiences, maintaining their interest throughout the session, and enabling players to remain highly attuned to the meanings and understandings drawn from the inquiry.

SUMMARY

Representation: Communicating Research Processes and Outcomes

This chapter presents three main formats for presenting the outcomes of research: *written reports*, *presentations*, and *performances*.

These provide evocative accounts enabling empathetic understanding of participant experience. They should:

- **Clearly and accurately *represent* participant *experiences* and *perspectives***
- **Be constructed to suit specific *audiences* and *purposes***

Written reports* may take the form of *accounts* and *narratives*, *biographies* or *ethnographies*, written as individual, joint, or collective accounts. They may take the form of *informal summary reports

for project participants, *formal reports* for professional and administrative audiences, or *academic reports* for research journals.

Presentations may integrate *a variety of media*, including verbal reports, charts, flow charts, maps, concept maps, art, figures, overheads, audio tapes, video, and electronic presentations.

Performances may include *drama, art, poetry, music*, or other formats. These may be stored, displayed, and presented in a variety of visual, oral, and electronic forms.

Procedures for constructing *written reports*, or *scripts*, for presentations and performances include:

- Identifying *audience* and *purpose*
- Selecting participant *perspectives*
- Reviewing the *data*
- Selecting *key features* and *elements* of experience from the analyzed data
- Constructing a *framework/outline* using these features
- *Writing* the report/script
- *Reviewing* and *editing* the report/script
- *Member checking* for accuracy and appropriateness

Taking Action: Passion, Purposes, and Pathways

RESEARCH DESIGN	DATA GATHERING	DATA ANALYSIS	REPRESENTATION	ACTION
INITIATING A STUDY	CAPTURING STAKEHOLDER EXPERIENCES AND PERSPECTIVES	IDENTIFYING KEY FEATURES OF EXPERIENCE	WRITING REPORTS	CREATING SOLUTIONS
Setting the stage			Reports Ethnographies Biographies	Care plans
Focusing and framing	Interviewing	Analyzing epiphanies and illuminative experiences	PRESENTATIONS AND PERFORMANCES	Case management
Literature review	Observing			Problem-solving
Stakeholders	Reviewing artifacts	Categorizing and coding	Presentations Drama Poetry	Enhancing practices
Data sources	Reviewing literature	Enhancing analysis	Song Dance Art	Evaluation
Ethics		Constructing category frameworks	Video Multimedia	Health promotion
Validity				Community development
				Professional development
				Strategic planning

Contents of This Chapter

This chapter describes ways to use the outcomes of data analysis to devise systematic actions to resolve problems and issues on which research has focused. It describes how to:
- Formulate and monitor *client care plans* using a multi-disciplinary *case-management* approach
- Establish mutual support groups for clients to develop *self-care strategies*
- Develop action plans for problem-solving processes
- *Enhance professional practices*

The chapter also describes how action research may be used for evaluation. Three models are presented:
- Open inquiry
- Collaborative evaluation
- Audit review evaluation

Action research is also presented as a method for formulating and implementing:
- Health promotion programs
- Community development
- Professional development programs
- Strategic planning for institutions, organizations, and agencies in the health sector

Introduction

The Act phase of the Look-Think-Act cycle of action research applies the knowledge and understandings emerging from research inquiry to immediate practical purposes—resolution of the research problem or issue. The next step, therefore, is an important transition from essentially reflective and communicative processes to practical actions that enable researchers to achieve the purposes of their inquiry. It is here where "the rubber meets the road," where health professionals take specific actions to improve client care practices or implement innovative health promotion strategies. Action research is applicable to individual clinical care, case management, primary health care, and health promotion programs focused on family and community groups.

The types of action emerging from these processes provide a particularly useful way for health practitioners to incorporate the principles of the Alma Ata Declaration on Primary Health Care (PHC), "Health for All" (UNICEF, 1978), and the directives of the Ottawa Charter on Health Promotion (Wass, 2000). By engaging both health service providers and recipients, practitioners establish a foundation for health care that is practical, socially and culturally acceptable, collaborative and accessible, and that encourages self-reliance and self-determination—all cardinal principles of PHC.

The Look-Think-Act cycle signals that research participants will use new understandings emerging from data analysis to enhance or change their work practices—to take appropriate "action" (see Figure 7.1).

Action research is particularly useful as a tool of inquiry for developing innovative solutions to a wide range of primary health care problems. This does not, however, encompass its full potential as a tool of inquiry. Many regular professional tasks—the development of care plans, care coordination, case management, health education, and health promotion interventions—may be greatly strengthened by the

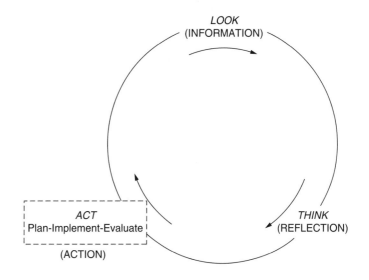

Figure 7.1
Taking Action

conscious application of systematic and participatory processes of inquiry. Individual care plans, family and community-based interventions, and associated professional practices require constant review as understandings and circumstances shift and new information emerges.

Engaging People's Passion

The process of healing and caring for others—central to the experience of health professionals—is complex, compelling, and often rewarding. Meaningful interventions require practitioners to bring their passion, creativity, and skills to the complex physical, social, cultural, moral, and spiritual dimensions of illness and well-being. The Action phase of the research cycle, therefore, provides considerable scope for health professionals to creatively engage in innovative and effective intervention strategies that engage the unique understandings and meanings clients bring to their own healing.

> As a primary health care practitioner, I recall the commitment and passion of people whose dedication enabled them to develop powerful solutions to public health problems in their small communities. They worked to build a shared understanding of the local situation with other residents and to identify and take ownership of health issues with them. Using participatory problem solving and planning processes, residents were able to develop innovative and successful solutions to community health problems. The service, commitment, and passion of local people who engage in this work is often awe-inspiring. Frequently, the relationships established within these challenging and inspiring projects have endured beyond the life of the project itself.

When taking action, we need to continue engaging the working principles of action research presented in Chapter 2:

- **Relationships:** Maintaining positive working relationships with all stakeholders
- **Communication:** Informing stakeholders of ongoing activities
- **Participation:** Providing opportunities for stakeholders to engage in worthwhile activities
- **Inclusion:** Including all stakeholders and all relevant issues

A key feature of this process is the need to ensure that primary stakeholders—those principally affected by the issue—are centrally involved in the process. By doing so, we acknowledge their competence and worth and engender high degrees of motivation and ownership that are the hallmarks of effective work practices.

The Nursing Process and Client Care

Specific components of action research directly parallel the key components of both the family physician's **Patient-Centred Clinical Method** (McWhinney, 1989) and the **Nursing Process** (Iyer, Tapitch, & Bernocchi-Losey, 1991). Both frameworks incorporate a process that may be seen to parallel the phases of action research: Look—client assessment and examination; Think—analysis and planning; and Act—implementation of care plans. Evaluation of these actions is achieved through the next cycle of the Look-Think-Act process.

These processes provide rich possibilities for the development and monitoring of innovative care solutions and the engagement of clients in self-management strategies that increase both their control of the healing process and its effectiveness. This is particularly the case when nursing plans or medical plans are incorporated as components of a multi-disciplinary action plan (MAP) (Cohen & Casta, 1993), and can inform processes of Continuous Quality Improvement (CQI) relating to care management.

Regular forums facilitated by the primary nurse practitioner in the nursing case-management role or the family physician in the care coordination role, with the participation of the client and other key, multi-disciplinary health providers, enables all involved to systematically acquire and review information relevant to the client. Such a process enables the collaborative development of specific, agreed upon, and individually appropriate care-management strategies.

A patient-centered clinical method or nursing process includes:

- Needs assessment (observation of diagnostic cues)
- Analysis (or diagnosis)
- Planning for care management
- Implementation of the care-management strategy
- Evaluation of the care plan

Assessment

In this phase of the action research cycle, health professionals and clients share their experience, knowledge, and interpretations of the problem. Health professionals bring an assessment of the relevant clinical, behavioral, and contextual cues from observations and physical examinations. The multi-disciplinary forum provides the opportunity for all data and associated issues and factors in the client's condition to be examined.

Analysis (or Diagnosis)

This equates with the Think phase of the action research cycle. The nursing case manager or physician coordinating care seeks to facilitate the development of a shared understanding by all participants in the case—a management forum of key diagnostic issues requiring intervention relevant to the healing of the client.

Planning

Planning also equates with Think—determining the priorities and desired outcomes, and developing a care plan, case-management plan, or multi-disciplinary action plan (MAP). A MAP will include some procedures that are already the subject of specific protocols. A key issue for the case manager is writing a plan in such a way that it is comprehensible by both the client and other health professionals responsible for client care.

Pathways of inquiry in the development of a *care plan* include:

- **Goal:** What outcome can the client realistically accomplish? What is the goal or purpose to be achieved?
- **Objectives:** What would the client and the health professionals involved need to do to achieve this goal/purpose? What are the priorities amongst these objectives? How can these objectives be documented, monitored, and evaluated?
- **Information/Skills:** What professional interventions are required? What knowledge and/or skills would the health professionals and the client need in order to accomplish the objectives? How would the health professional or the client acquire these skills and knowledge?
- **Resources:** What resources or materials are needed by either the health professional or the client? How can these be made available?
- **Networks:** Who else can be involved in patient management and care? Who is available to provide the emotional support to a client attempting to manage their own self-care?
- **Accountability:** Who is the designated case manager, and what pathways are available to them to ensure that other health professionals work within the guidelines?

The process presented in the section on Action Planning, which follows, may assist the development of a care plan.

Implementation

Implementation engages the Act phase of the research cycle—implementing the various facets of a multi-disciplinary action plan. These will include the nursing plan and the medical plan and their prescribed regimens of care. A key responsibility of the case manager or care coordinator is to coordinate services and providers and supervision of client care. This will also entail ensuring that clients have access to necessary resources, fostering the maintenance of a healing environment, linking clients with specialist services, and providing advocacy where required. Often, a one-page summary of the MAP or a "critical path" provides the basis for implementation and review.

Evaluation

Evaluation engages the next cycle of the action research process—Look-Think-Act. The health professionals and the client gather information for the purpose of reviewing the enactment of the MAP, discovering what is working well, identifying what requires change, and deciding what needs to work more effectively. Again, the participation of the case manager, other key professionals, and the client or their representative adds greater dimension to the case management review process. They are able to bring their experience, knowledge, unique understandings, and meanings to examine implementation processes, analyzing reasons for variation in the case-management plan and deciding how things could be done differently.

Action research, therefore, provides a way for multi-disciplinary case management teams to position inquiry centrally and consciously within their practice. Not only does it enable them to document a unique account of the immediate task at hand, but it also makes use of accounts of innovative strategies available in the literature.

Case Management: Managing Chronic Illness

Recent research (Dodds, 1995; Koch, Kralik, Eastwood, & Schofield, 2001; Koch, Selim, & Kralik, 2002) describes how action research can enhance the management of chronic illness. Community nurse practitioners operating from a large community nursing organization have undertaken action research projects to assist their clients live with and manage chronic illness, including diabetes and multiple sclerosis (Koch, Kralik, Eastwood, & Schofield, 2001; Koch, Kralik, & Kelly, 2000; Koch, Kralik, & Sonnack, 2000; Koch, Kralik, & Taylor, 2000.)

They have adapted the Look-Think-Act action research cycle documented by Stringer (1999):

- **Looking** means gathering information, defining and describing the situation, and constructing a preliminary understanding of the context (Koch, Selim, & Kralik, 2002). This phase of the inquiry enables participants to share their experiences of living with their disease. It also allows health professionals to share their professional insights.
- **Thinking** refers to exploring, analyzing, interpreting, and explaining. Participants discuss their experiences (data gathering) and identify emergent themes (data analysis).
- **Acting** refers to the development, implementation, and evaluation of plans devised by the participants. Individual participants develop new strategies to improve their self-management, their ability to cope with the disease in general, and their ability to enhance their self-esteem. Collectively, they can support each other in gaining access to community services and appropriate products.

Enhancing Workplace Practices

Action research provides health managers with a framework to apply systematic inquiry to the development of quality workplace practices. On-site, participatory inquiry enables practitioners to develop unique and specific practice protocols tailored to the context of a particular health service team or organization. Examples include improvements to wound care management (Koch, Selim, & Kralik, 2002), prevention of workplace violence within nursing settings (Koch, Selim, & Kralik, 2000), changes to midwifery practices in a women's hospital (Barrett, 2001), and the documentation and benchmarking of health worker practices (Genat, 2001).

Tina Koch and her colleagues (Koch, Selim, & Kralik, 2002) adopted a participatory action research framework inspired by Street (1995), similar to the Look-Think-Act cycle outlined in this book. The steps undertaken in their investigation include:

- **Reconnaissance or preliminary investigation:** Collaborative research and review of the current literature into wound management (Look)
- **Research question or problem identification:** Identify specific issues for investigation. In this example, nurses explored best practice protocols for cleansing chronic leg ulcers (Think)
- **Plan for action:** Develop a shared strategy for implementing and monitoring practice (Act)
- **Taking action and collecting data on action:** Participants consciously reflect on their practice and share their knowledge and practice reflections with colleagues (Act and Look)
- **Analyze data:** Participants collectively identify key elements of their practice (Think)
- **Reflect:** Participants develop a rationale for practice (Think)
- **Re-plan, reflect, and so on:** Continue to monitor implementation of the protocol (Act-Look-Think)

A similar practice framework adopted by Penelope Barrett (2001) was directed towards improving midwifery practice and enhancing women's satisfaction with their early mothering experiences. The process included:

- **Collaborating** throughout the project with midwives in clinical practice at a women's hospital
- **Identifying concerns** related to women's experiences of informed choice during the early mothering period *(Look)*
- **Prioritizing** these concerns and identifying a thematic concern/substantive problem related to the practice *(Think)*
- **Developing a plan** of critically informed action to address the thematic concern and improve what is happening *(Act)*
- **Observing the effects** of the critically informed action within the context in which it occurs *(Look)*
- **Reflecting on and evaluating these effects** as a basis for further planning *(Think)*

By placing inquiry at the heart of the process, health professionals are able to share and refine their existing practice knowledge in collaboration with their colleagues.

Problem Solving: Action Planning

Solutions to emerging issues often require careful planning to ensure successful resolution of a problem. The following section delineates a simple action planning process.

Setting Priorities: Establishing an Action Agenda

Having engaged in data collection or needs assessment and analysis, participants will review information and identify key issues to be addressed. From these, they will construct a set of agendas upon which they will take action.

Participants will:

- Review the needs assessment *focus*, *question*, and *objectives*
- Review the framework of *issues*, *key features*, and *elements* emerging from data analysis
- From these select *agendas* requiring action
- *Prioritize* the issues, distinguishing those requiring immediate action from those which may be handled in the medium or long term

Creating Pathways: Constructing an Action Plan

Carefully formulated plans enable research participants to envision the concrete steps needed to accomplish a desired outcome. Participants devise action plans for each agenda item. Each plan will include:

- **Why:** A statement of overall *purpose*
- **What:** A set of *objectives* to be attained
- **How:** A sequence of *tasks* and *steps* for each objective
- **Who:** The *people* responsible for each task and activity
- **Where:** The *place* where the tasks will be done
- **When:** The *time* when tasks should commence and be completed

The plan should include arrangements to monitor and support people as they enact their tasks.

Some of our colleagues were involved in a project focusing on "the lack of support services for the frail-aged." Participants restated the issue as a *goal*:

- To increase support services for the frail-aged.

Reviewing the analysis from previous phases of research revealed factors related to lack of support services for the frail-aged. These included:

- Lack of transport
- Limited access to prepared meals
- Unhealthy living conditions

These were restated as three objectives:

- To develop a transport service
- To organize access to meals-on-wheels
- To organize an in-home cleaning service

> Teams of relevant stakeholders, including frail-aged people and their family members, community health nurses, social workers, and members of other support programs developed a plan for each issue and brought them to a combined planning session for discussion, modification, and endorsement of all stakeholders. In this case, each planning group included a member from each of the primary stakeholding groups, including the frailaged.

A planning chart may be used to clearly articulate all facets of the work (see Figure 7.2).

Reviewing the Plan

When details have been entered on the chart, participants can review the plan to check and clarify each person's responsibilities, the sequence of activities, and materials and resources required for each task:

- Have all needed materials and/or equipment been identified? Who will obtain them? Where from? When?

PURPOSE (Why): What are we trying to achieve?							
OBJECTIVE What	TASKS How	PERSON(S) Who	START When	FINISH	LOCATION Where	RESOURCES	FUNDS
1. Provide a transport service to the frail-aged	a) Determine frail-aged eligibility for subsidized taxi service-access research funds	Mr. Whipple Ms. Jones Rotary volunteers	6.3.02	8.5.02	Survey in frail-aged own homes	Time Survey forms Volunteers	Seeding grant to research frail-aged needs $3000
	b) Brief local taxi drivers on recoup of taxi vouchers	Ms. Jones	7.4.02	8.5.02	Taxi Depot	Time Taxi voucher guidelines	
	c) Bus submission to federal aged care program	Rotary Club Chair Jenny	6.3.02	7.4.02	Rotary Club Premises	Funding guidelines Survey results	
2. Enable the frail-aged access to meals on wheels	a) Establish the need	Bruce Jose	6.3.02	7.4.02	Survey in frail-aged own homes	Time Survey forms Volunteers	
	b) Access funding guidelines	Venus Jose	6.3.02	7.4.02	Own offices	Telephone	
	c) Develop a submission	Bruce Jose Venus	7.4.02	8.5.02	Community Health Center	Survey results Historical data Endorsement from community leadership	

Figure 7.2
Planning Chart

- Are funds needed? Where will they come from? Who will organize them? When?
- Do people have adequate time to accomplish their tasks?
- Should other people be involved? For what tasks?
- Who will ask them? How will they become part of the process?
- Who will describe the project to them?
- How can they become part of our community?

Each of these elements is included in the review of the plan, with objectives, tasks, and activities carefully defined and assigned. Larger or more complex issues may require monitoring an extensive array of activities, but smaller projects usually need only limited time and resources for planning.

Sometimes planning procedures become stalled because people focus on emerging difficulties. Statements arise such as "What about . . . ," "Yes, but we can't do this because . . . ," "The director won't allow . . . ," "Clients can't . . . ," "Family members aren't capable of . . . ," "We haven't the time to . . . ," "The funds aren't available to . . . ," and so on. If these statements are left unanswered, people will soon become de-energized and an air of futility will result.

These types of concerns need to be formally acknowledged, clearly recorded, and incorporated into the planning process. It is essential that these issues be seen as problems to be solved, rather than reasons not to take action. Each should be reformulated from a **problem** to a statement of an *objective or task*, which is entered into the action plan. The problem "Funds aren't available," for instance, might be formulated as an objective "To seek an funds from. . . ," or "To search for sources of funding for . . . from . . ." This objective would be extrapolated through *tasks and activities*, a *person* responsible for the tasks, and a *time-line* for beginning and completing the tasks.

Supervision: Supporting and Monitoring Progress

Participants should designate a person to supervise the implementation of the plan. The designated person will check with people to learn whether they are able to carry out their tasks in the time allocated and to assist them to work through minor problems. The person supervising will communicate with participants regularly, using informal conversations in lunch rooms, outside of case meetings or other common meeting places, or by phone messages or email. In monitoring progress, the supervising person should also see themselves as offering personal support, especially for people working in difficult situations or carrying out difficult or complex tasks. Often, in these situations, they merely need to be a "listening ear," providing a means for participants to debrief, vent where necessary, or review the work they're doing.

Progress should also be monitored at meetings of participants. These should be regular enough to ensure that people remain committed to the project and to each other. Meetings should provide opportunities for people to report on their activities, review the overall plan, make any modifications or changes in objectives and tasks, and celebrate successes.

Evaluation: Assessing the Value and Quality of Programs and Services

This section presents three models of program evaluation concomitant with participatory action research: open inquiry evaluation, audit review evaluation (Wadsworth 1997), and collaborative evaluation (Maltrud, Polacsek, & Wallerstein, 1997). Readers engaged in the evaluation of large and complex projects would do well to consult these sources in detail.

Everyday Evaluation on the Run

Yoland Wadsworth (1997) presents two approaches to evaluation applicable to health programs—open inquiry evaluation and audit review evaluation. Like action research, Wadsworth's approach to evaluation works through reiterative processes of inquiry enabling participants to jointly explore their work, gain greater insight into their activities, and identify ways to solve problems or enhance the outcomes they seek. Participants build or extend their common understandings of the worth of their activities and test the value of what they are achieving.

Open Inquiry Evaluation

Key steps in this approach to evaluation include:

- **Reflection:** Enabling program participants to review collectively their own actions in the world and reflect upon their experience. Reflective questions may include:
  - **General questions:** How are we going? What are we doing? What's working? What's not? How do we know?
  - **Problem-posing and problem-solving questions:** How could we improve things?
  - **Needs:** What are the customer or client needs?
  - **"Opening up" questions:** Why are we doing this?
  - **Problems:** What are obvious and immediate problems?
  - **Assumptions and intentions:** What are people's underlying assumptions and intentions?
  - **Evaluation criteria:** Interrogating existing evaluation criteria.
- **"Design:"** Naming" the issue or problem and systematically answering questions arising, such as:
  - Who or what is to be researched?
  - Who will be the researchers?
  - Who is it for?
  - Whose lives will be improved?

- **Fieldwork:** Enabling all relevant parties to reach an effective understanding of what different people think, value, and what things mean to them.
- **Analysis and conclusions:** Identify themes, trends, or understandings to develop conclusions, explanations, and theories.
- **Feedback:** Check with the participants that the evaluation process got it right and that findings are understandable, plausible, or convincing.
- **Planning:** Realistic, practical, and achievable recommendations for change and improved practice are prioritized, planned, and put into practice.

An open inquiry approach to evaluation, through its focus on identifying and solving problems, increases the chances of improving health programs and services. It enables innovative, creative, and dynamic ideas and perspectives to emerge and provides participants with a sense of enthusiasm.

Audit Review Evaluation

The sense of this approach is signaled by the word "audit"—to check. The audit starts with different questions and has different endpoints. The audit review focuses on:

- **Objectives:** It starts with questions based on an existing set of objectives—Have we done what we set out to do? What are the signs we have done this?
- **Gaps and irrelevancies:** It asks questions about gaps and irrelevancies—What are we not doing? What are we doing that we shouldn't?
- **Needs:** Assumes community needs are known
- **Distills information:** The questions are narrowing down, checking activities on the bases of pre-existing understandings
- **Reveals problems:** Systematically problematizes all existing activities (i.e., checks to see if they are problematic)
- **Reviews practices:** Examines practices in light of existing objectives

An audit review has the advantage of checking all matters previously planned for, reassuring participants that much has been done, and matters not yet attended to will be attended to. The comprehensive nature of this approach is especially advantageous if the prior research base was strong, enabling participants to affirm previous agreements and strengthening a collective sense of direction. The fixed nature of the exploration also can feel very comfortable, providing a sense of stability and unity.

The audit review, however, does not always discriminate between still-valuable activities and those that have become outdated. It does not identify what needs to change or how changes might be accomplished. The attention to detail enabling a comprehensive review of activity may also be tedious and wastefully time-consuming.

Participatory Evaluation

Maltrud, Polacsek, and Wallerstein (1997)[1] have applied a participatory approach to a wide range of health programs and health initiatives. Evaluation is assumed to be an integral part of all facets of program development and implementation. It includes:

- A shared process
- Capacity building
- Feedback and reflection
- Involvement of different stakeholders

According to the authors, evaluation is important because it enables people to:

- Reflect on their progress
- Determine if they are doing what they set out to do
- Sustain their work over time
- Access decision makers and policymakers
- Share and support each other
- Develop inter-sectoral links with other private and public agencies that generate health impacts
- Celebrate their accomplishments

Steps in Collaborative Evaluation

The following framework provides an outline of the steps for an evaluation process. Each step, however, requires a range of activities needed to accomplish that part of the evaluation process. Each might be seen as an iteration of an action research cycle. Details for accomplishing each step are described by the authors in their handbook.

- **Sharing histories:** Participants tell stories that enable them to develop a unique history of the initiative. It enables them to create a common purpose for all members, to exchange information and correct misinformation, to identify deep-seated interests and values they have in common, to honor past accomplishments, and to build on existing efforts.
- **Creating a common vision:** A vision or mission statement describes a long-term, ideal, healthy community. It provides a common aspiration and enables people to see where they are going.
- **Identifying evaluation stakeholders:** The evaluation should include people who have a special or specific interest in the project. They may include community leaders, program staff, advocacy groups, state agencies, and community members. Stakeholders may also include evaluators or researchers, program directors, funding agencies, or policymakers.

---

[1]Copies of the Community Evaluation Workbook for Community Initiatives are available from: Nina Wallerstein, Masters in Public Health Program, 2400 Tucker NE, University of New Mexico School of Medicine, Albuquerque, NM 87131-5267.

- **Negotiating and identifying evaluand indicators and targets/objectives:** Deciding on the "evaluand"—that which is to be evaluated—is key to the health evaluation project. Evaluand indicators are categories of change that will be measured over time. Targets/objectives describe changes to be achieved as a result of health program activities. These are described in terms of outcomes, benchmarks, milestones, and performance measures. The process for identifying evaluand indicators and targets/objectives includes:
  - Choosing an *issue* (to identify the evaluand) as a starting point
  - Conducting an analysis of *causes* and *resources* related to the issue
  - Identifying *system* indicators and targets/objectives related to the issue (policies, community participation, organizations, resources, programs and services, etc.)
  - Identifying *population/people* indicators and targets/objectives related to the issue (knowledge, behavior, attitudes, health status, etc.)
  - Identifying *process* indicators and targets—the type activities and strategies that can be used to accomplish objectives
  - Use *logs* to chart progress towards each target
- **Plan strategies:** Participants define the strategies they will use to reach the targets/objectives, incorporating evaluation as an ongoing part of the planning, implementation, and evaluation phases of the ongoing project.
- **Track the indicators and collect data:** Participants gather information to chart their progress, beginning with baseline data that enables them to know where they started. Subsequently, they collect primary and secondary data related to identified targets/objectives.
- **Analyze data:** Suggested approaches to data analysis include:
  - Comparing baseline data with a similar population
  - Comparing baseline data to state data
  - Comparing initiative data over time (e.g., annually)
  - Creating visual ways to describe what is happening
- **Communicate evaluation results:** The authors emphasize the importance of sharing results at different points in the process to get the word out about what has been discovered. Short-term and long-term outcomes can be shared with others as preliminary or final reports. Results should be widely shared with initiative members, community and political leaders, other community groups, state programs and initiatives, and funding sources. Reports and presentations should be simple, clear, and attractive.

Community Development

More recent approaches to public health have their origins in the Alma-Ata Declaration on Primary Health Care (World Health Organization, 1988) and the Ottawa Charter on Health Promotion (World Health Organization, 1986), which recognize that health and illness are embedded in social and cultural contexts. They also recognize that not all sectors of the community attribute the same meanings to health matters. In these circumstances, community development provides strategies for participants to rebuild supportive networks and relationships, to empower local interest groups within the public arena, and to incorporate local social and cultural meanings and understandings into program development.

The practice of community development in health begins with a group of people gathering together for the purpose of addressing a common health concern:

> In the term "community development" the word "community" refers to a local or identifiable *community of interest*. . . community development means the development of that community or network. . . internally in terms of its coherence and consciousness of itself (*identity*), and externally, in terms of that group's power in relation to structures of broader society (*empowerment*). (our italics) (CDIH, 1988, p. 10)

Community development focuses on a small, local group establishing:

- Its own coherence, solidarity, and common vision
- Partnerships with other local community and professional groups

Butler and Cass (1993) present community development processes in the following terms:

- **Control of decision-making:** Community members participate to control the project and particularly to control the identification and definition of the issue
- **Involvement in the action:** The project involves the people concerned with the issue in action for change
- **Development of community culture:** The project contributes to a culture of groups of individuals taking responsibility for improving and protecting their areas and services
- **Organizational development:** The project builds a new organization or improves an existing one
- **Learning:** The participants acquire new skills, information, and/or new perspectives on themselves, their community, and their concerns
- **Concrete benefit:** The project sees the achievement of some new or improved service or facility, or the protection of something valued by the community
- **New power relationships:** The project changes the social landscape of the community so that new and more equitable power relations are formed

The Community Development in Health Project (1988) identified two strategies for facilitating community development projects. These strategies (somewhat adapted) include *consensus building strategies* and *empowerment strategies*. One can chart clear parallels here between the strategies of community development in health and action research as it has been described in previous chapters.

Consensus Building Strategies

The main features of consensus building strategies include:

- **Strengthening empathy and trust:** These are developed both with and amongst participants by:

- Using a relaxed style of communication
- Ensuring participants are comfortable in the environment
- Enabling participants to relate their experiences freely with each other
- **Building a shared picture:** Gathering participant perspectives concerning the issues or problems under investigation. By encouraging all participants to share their experience, the research facilitator or community development worker assists participants to identify common experiences and perceptions. Discrepancies between participant experiences are often an entry point for further inquiry and potentially provide all participants with a deeper contextual understanding of the issue at hand.
- **Working together:** By undertaking a collective, shared task (designing the project, collecting data, analyzing data, and presenting findings), participants build empathy and trust, appreciate each other's strengths and foibles, and strengthen their relationships. The solidarity built through this process can sustain groups when other stakeholders question their perceptions, are unwilling to acknowledge their findings, or challenge their recommendations.

Empowerment Strategies

Empowerment strategies are characterized by:

- **Information:** A community development project requires participants to acquire and share information, establish contacts to solicit further information, and engage in archival research. These activities enable participants to become better informed and acquire an extensive understanding of the issues under inquiry.
- **Relationships—building links and partnerships:** Build relationships both internally within the primary group identified as the community of interest and externally with other local and regional stakeholders including those within relevant organizations and institutions. External relationships link the primary reference group with other like-minded groups, with sympathizers within the health bureaucracy, and with influential businesses and organizations.
- **Decision-making:** Participants control decision-making through their participation in research design, appropriate data gathering and analysis methods, and constructing representations.
- **Consciousness raising—building a broader awareness:** Consumers build a greater awareness of factors affecting their health through the social learning component of action research, enabling participants to recognize new ways to resolve particular problems. This also provides a basis for consciousness-raising in the broader community through the dissemination of information derived from action research processes.

In summary, community development and action research share significant similarities in both methods and outcome. Action research, as outlined in the previous chapters, provides community development practitioners with powerful ways to capture the insights revealed within the "social learning" component of their practice.

By finding skillful ways to record local narratives using the idiosyncratic language and shared everyday meanings that people bring to their understandings of local health issues, action research processes can strengthen and enhance community development processes.

Developing Health Promotion Programs

The underlying premise of health promotion, according to the World Health Organization (1986), suggests that "to reach a state of complete physical, mental, and social well-being, an individual or group must be able to identify and to realize aspirations, to satisfy needs, and to change or cope with the environment." Action research is an effective way to build healthy public policy, create supportive environments, strengthen community action, develop personal skills, and to re-orient health services—the five imperatives of the Ottawa Charter on Health Promotion.

Action research methods complement health promotion because as Green (1992) suggests "public health education begins 'where the people are' as a matter of principle and because educational research, especially on adult populations, has demonstrated that the commitment of people to the goals of a program increases the probability of their participation, co-operation, or behavioral response to a program." A common practice framework for developing and implementing small-scale health promotion programs includes the following steps:

- Assess needs
- Prioritize issues or needs
- Plan
- Implement the health promotion program
- Evaluate and reassesss

Health professionals should be certain that local people recognize the importance of ensuring that the diversity of groupings within the community are incorporated into the project. Local communities comprise a diverse range of ethnic, gender, age, and other interest-defined groups. It is necessary to identify all key stakeholders and either gain their direct participation or keep them fully informed. This is particularly crucial in the planning phase of the project.

Needs Assessment

Needs assessment can be informed by:

- Client or consumer perspectives on crucial and significant factors affecting their health
- Epidemiological surveys of relationships between the incidence of disease and exposure to potential risk factors
- Knowledge, attitude, and belief (KAB) surveys
- Local research reports

Where needs are predetermined by existing information categories, a program may omit or distort crucial information derived from the knowledge of local people.

Prioritize Needs

Whereas a health planner may read a set of incidence rates for particular diseases and decide a need exists for a health promotion intervention, the residents in the location may determine health intervention needs on the basis of a different, more context-specific set of values.

In order to prioritize needs, the health professional would undertake the following key steps:

- Facilitate processes for local people to share their *health concerns*
- Assist them to develop a *collective picture* of current health issues in their own community
- Have them formulate a picture or *vision* of their community in more ideal, healthier terms
- On the basis of the vision, examine local health problems and their *predisposing, reinforcing, and enabling* factors
- On the basis of the vision, *prioritize* locally driven health interventions

Local people should develop a collective picture of the current state of their own community health, their vision for a healthier community, and, on that basis, the health priorities that require intervention. By facilitating such processes and standing alongside people as a collaborator and consultant, practitioners can develop significant levels of local support for health promotion interventions.

Planning

It is during the planning phase of the project, where local people have decided to focus on a specific health intervention, that clear recognition of the key stakeholders is crucial. In particular, it is necessary to clearly decide which community groups will be the intended, direct beneficiaries of the project—the primary reference groups (PRG). In order for project planning to be effective, it is important that representatives of the PRG and other key stakeholders are included.

Stakeholding groups will:

- Determine objectives
- Define strategies
- Decide who will undertake particular tasks
- Identify the resources required to complete these tasks
- Develop an inventory of local assets
- Arrange access to existing community assets and resources

While resources may already exist in the community that could assist the project, exisiting divisions between groups in the community may prevent access. Likewise, the availability of particular specific skills and expertise, information, networks, contacts, and power and influence will depend on who is involved in the project.

Implementation

During the implementation phase, the health professional will:

- Convene regular reviews of progress with the local participants

- Report on their experiences, which should be completed by all stakeholders, including and especially the PRG
- Document progress and emerging problems
- Celebrate successes
- Devise solutions to problems

Within a well-developed project, the local facilitator and members of the steering group will have extensive backup networks and resources for troubleshooting when particular facets of the plan strike trouble. In the implementation phase of the project, it will not always be possible for the health professional and local project steering group to *all* meet to resolve issues. A key consideration, as indicated in Chapter 3, is to ensure that these processes are public.

Evaluation

At this stage, it may be useful to convene a forum that includes people from all stakeholder groups to hear about the outcomes of their work and share their experiences. They should:

- Review objectives, strategies
- Review tasks completed
- Review tasks to be completed
- Describe outcomes of tasks completed
- Match these outcomes to the objectives
- Identify successful accomplishments
- Identify gaps—points where tasks have not been completed or objectives have not been attained
- Celebrate successes
- Review objectives, strategies, and tasks

Action research adds a highly significant dimension to the implementation of health promotion projects. The systematic methods outlined in the preceding chapters provide powerful ways to make a difference.

Professional Development: Collaborative Reflective Practice

Action research provides an effective tool for integrating quality assurance and "best practice" inquiry methods into specific components of professional development. Stein, Smith, and Silver (1999) suggest effective professional development processes have the following characteristics:

- **On-site development:** Development and implementation of the program within the professional work environment
- **Organizational resource allocation:** Including, time, space, and expertise
- **A learning community:** Conscious strategies directed toward the development of a practice-based learning community
- **Active networks:** Valuing and utilizing existing links to appropriate people and organizational resources in the community

- **Integration with strategic plans:** Areas of professional development are linked to organizational plans

Systematic processes of action research enhance the design and implementation of an effective program of professional development. The research framework presented in this book provides a resource enabling health professionals to:

- Identify professional development needs
- Identify issues related to those needs—specific health discipline standards, technological advances, managerial imperatives, and so on.
- Set goals/objectives for professional development
- Plan strategies of professional development
- Implement and evaluate professional development strategies

Systematic process of inquiry will enable health administrators to build professional development activities into ongoing programs, drawing on the experience and wisdom of their existing staff, and identifying ways to access other sources of expertise. Through processes of reflection and dialogue inherent in action research, they can work with colleagues and other stakeholders to explore the following questions:

- What are their current strengths?
- What are the problematic issues in their work?
- What is to be learned by whom?
- How will these things be learned?
- Who will facilitate and support the learning process?
- Who will provide expertise?
- How will time and resources be allocated?
- How will new learning be supported, reinforced, and extended?
- How will new learning be assessed and reviewed?
- What financial resources will be allocated?

The alignment of training and development with existing federal, state, and regional health plans and seamless integration with the corporate plan of the organization will further enhance professional development programs.

Strategic Planning: Building the Big Picture

Although action research is often associated with small scale, local studies, it is a viable tool that may be applied to the management of large organizations. Action research may be used in the workplace for strategic planning at the team level, but is equally applicable to corporate planning within a "whole of organization approach" or to a state health system. The collaborative strategic planning processes that follow are implicit in Total Quality Management (Huffman, 1997; Tennant 2001), but are also relevant to more generalized processes of planning and administration (Block, 1990; Coughlan & Brannick, 2001). Action research processes enable health administrators to systematically gather and analyze the large volume of information necessary to produce effective strategic plans that are in touch with the people.

Vision Statements

Health organizations and state health systems describe the "big picture" of their healing intent within policy documents incorporating *vision* and *mission* statements that are the manifestations of an underlying philosophy on health care. They include broad statements of *purpose* and *value* defining a philosophy of health service provision. Such statements may cover fundamental issues related to democratic social and community life, and underlying moral and ethical principles. An example of a vision statement is provided by The Declaration of Alma Ata that was subsequently endorsed by the World Health Organization (1978):

> Health, which is a state of complete physical, mental, and social well being, and not merely the absence of disease or infirmity, is a fundamental human right and that the attainment of the highest possible level of health is a most important world-wide social goal whose realization requires the action of many other social and economic sectors in addition to the health sector.
>
> Governments have a responsibility for the health of their people which can be fulfilled only by the provision of adequate health and social measures. A main social target of governments, international organizations, and the whole world community in the coming decades should be the attainment by all peoples of the world by the year 2000 of a level of health that will permit them to lead a socially and economically productive life. Primary health care is a key to attaining this target as part of development in the spirit of social justice.

Vision statements guiding health policy within ministries of health in many countries have since incorporated similar values and purposes. A coherent policy should provide strong degrees of association between broad policy statements and particular health programs enacted through all levels of the system. Broad vision statements, which are essentially philosophical in nature, need to be specifically linked to particular programs, services, and educational activities. Carefully articulated links at each level of planning provide guidance for practitioners to move from *vision*, to *mission*, to *operational* and *action plans* detailing how these programs and services are to be instituted.

A local district health council may construct a vision for health through the following type of statement:

> *The Newbury District Health Service will provide quality health care for all Newbury citizens, regardless of race, ethnicity, class, gender, or sexual orientation, making provision for their physical, social, emotional, and spiritual well-being at all levels of the health system.*

Mission Statements

Mission statements describe how this vision is to be achieved. For example:

The Newbury District Health Service will:

- Provide accessible primary, secondary, and tertiary levels of care within an integrated service delivery system

- Design and implement appropriate health promotion programs for all identified client groups
- Provide special services for those most at risk (children from 0–5; young mothers; youth)
- Provide necessary management and administrative resources to ensure effective and timely delivery of services
- Provide necessary budgetary guidelines and financial resources sufficient to implement cost-effective programs and services

Operational Plans

The district would articulate an operational plan that describes a set of specific objectives related to each of these mission statements. For example:

The Newbury District Health Service will:

- Provide primary, secondary, and tertiary services health services from each of the clinics in the district
- Provide community-based services to frail-aged and disabled clients within the district
- Provide maternity services within the Southside Clinic
- Organize and coordinate the ongoing operation of those programs
- Link the agency effectively to clients, their families, and partner agencies in the community.
- Provide supervision and administrative support for those programs through the health service administration
- Provide resources—equipment and materials—and special services in support of the community-based service
- Evaluate the effectiveness of the service

Action Plans

Action plans provide step-by-step details of the ways in which each of the activities, services, or programs described in the operational plan will be put into practice. As they do so, they incorporate the values and principles enshrined in the mission statement, ensuring that programs and services reflect the broader intents of the planning process. These details can be formulated, reviewed, and evaluated using action research routines and provide the means for the integrated development of programs and services within the system. Opportunities for health teams to plan and review their work in this way provides the impetus for thinking outside the box, maintaining their focus on the real purposes of their endeavors, and enhancing their professional life.

The strategic planning process depicted in Figure 7.3 is a nominal version of an actual planning process. It shows the levels of planning that need to occur and

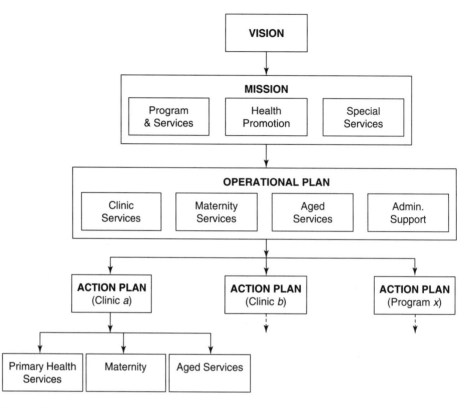

Figure 7.3
Strategic Planning Framework

signals the interconnection between the different sections. The figure illustrates how the provision of clinic and outreach services is linked to larger health and social issues and agendas. Action research provides the means for health professionals to systematically acquire and analyze the complex array of information required to formulate effective health programs and services.

SUMMARY

Taking Action: Passion, Purposes, and Pathways

This chapter outlines ways action research can be applied to common health frameworks to enhance the effectiveness of the professional practices:

The Nursing Process and Client Care
Case Management: Managing Chronic Illness

Enhancing Workplace Practices

Problem Solving: Action Planning

Evaluation: Assessing the Value and Quality of Health Programs and Services

Community Development

Developing Health Promotion Programs

Professional Development: Collaborative Reflective Practice

Strategic Planning: Building the Big Picture

Action Research in Health: Case Studies

8

Introduction

Examples of action research projects in clinics, hospitals, and other health contexts are proliferating rapidly. The extent of interest in this form of investigation is demonstrated by expanding audiences at action research sessions at conferences and reports in academic and professional journals. It is becoming a recognized tool of health professionals and an increasingly regular part of pre-service preparation and in-service professional development.

The following case studies, therefore, represent but a few of the creative and productive ways health professionals have applied action research in their work and community contexts. They are real-life studies, providing some indication of the diversity of forms taken by research methodologies similar to those described in this book. Each case differs in style and quality and does not necessarily represent best practice in action research. Some are not defined by the authors as action research, though they do represent its underlying processes and purposes or illustrate features of research processes presented in previous chapters. They include the following:

1. Self-Care Strategies in Community Nursing
2. Psychotherapy: Focusing Client Self-Help Groups
3. Health Promotion and Community Development: Hazardous Waste Problems
4. Creative Prevention Strategies: Hospitals and the Community
5. Primary Health Care: Investigating Alcohol Issues
6. Parent Participation and Involvement in the Care of a Hospitalized Child
7. Change Management in an Interdisciplinary In-patient Facility within Health Services
8. Incorporating the Social Context: Collaborative Reflection within a Family Practice
9. Developing Acute Care Protocols in Accident and Emergency
10. Integrating the Isolated Aged into Community Practice
11. Developing Clinical Protocols for Cataract Surgery
12. Action Research and Evidence-Based Wound Management
13. Collaborative Inquiry into a WHO Protocol: Stories of Family Physicians
14. The Oncology Clinic Tea Trolley: Community Development in Health
15. Entry to Cross-Cultural Inquiry: The House Party

1. Self-Care Strategies in Community Nursing

Tina Koch and Debbie Kralik, along with their colleagues in a large, urban community-nursing service, have incorporated action research into their practice to enhance both the lives of the clients and the services provided to them. Investigating experiences of living with chronic illnesses with their clients, they have been able to identify improved methods of providing care and assisting people to develop better self-care strategies. A recent focus of their work has been with clients who live with and manage diabetes and multiple sclerosis (Koch, Kralik, Eastwood, & Schofield, 2001; Koch, Kralik, & Kelly, 2000; Koch, Kralik, & Sonnack, 2000; Koch, Kralik, & Taylor, 2000).

One inquiry into incontinence (Koch, Kralik, Eastwood, & Schofield, 2001) involved four nursing consultants who assisted eight middle-class women living with multiple sclerosis to form a Participatory Action Research group. Because the primary research question concerned the ways that clients managed incontinence, the women living with the disease sought physiological information on how multiple sclerosis affected bladder function and shared information about everyday ways to manage their illness. The women investigated containment strategies, managing urinary tract infections, sexual relationships, engagement with health professionals, community services, and strategies for living well in the context of chronic illness.

Common themes emerging from this process included their lack of voice in the health system and the code of silence surrounding their illness, particularly concerning both incontinence and sexuality. They identified a shared difficulty in obtaining suitable containment products and a lack of appropriate community facilities for the disabled, focusing particularly on accessibility of toilets. Through dialogue, they validated each other's experiences, created shared meanings of the illness experience, and legitimated and strengthened their sense of self and identity. Particular difficulties and what were previously perceived as "peculiar" coping behaviours became "normalized" within the group.

The women were able to take action to implement, review, and refine alternative strategies to maintain their quality of life as they improved their ways of managing incontinence. In the process, they successfully petitioned the city council for better access to public toilet facilities and arranged for improved delivery systems of containment products with suppliers.

In summary, Koch and Kralik observe, "A person living with chronic illness may find him/herself in a nexus of dynamic events that may result in a loss of functioning, financial strain, family distress, personal distress, stigma and threats to former self-images. If health care professionals can understand the process that facilitates people to move towards incorporating chronic illness into their lives, we can make a substantial contribution to enhance their chronic disease, self-care management and their lives." (Koch & Kralick, 2001a).

2. Psychotherapy: Focusing Client Self-Help Groups

INTRODUCTION

In her healing work as a psychotherapist, Dr. Jacqui Dodds was both intrigued by and disturbed about the experiences she encountered amongst cancer patients who utilize alternative healing strategies alongside the biomedical treatments advocated by most oncologists. She describes one attraction of action research as the "emphasis on social change and collaboration and its pro-active, change-inducing goals" (Dodds, 1999: 43, 46). In a recent conversation, Dodds described both how and why she used participatory action research to investigate the experiences of cancer patients.

Prior to her project with cancer patients, Dodds provided counseling services within an organization dedicated to mutual support for cancer patients and their families. With the approval of the organization, she advertised her interest in working with a group of cancer patients to explore their experiences living with cancer. Subsequently, she facilitated three different "collaborative inquiry groups" through a cycle of 10 meetings.

FRAMING THE INQUIRY

Although familiar with survey research methods and quantitative analysis, Dodds observes, "Meanings that people make . . . of a human situation require a much more qualitative approach . . . if you set up all the questions yourself, you're completely setting the agenda—you can only get your information in relation to the questions that you've asked. This, invariably, leaves out interesting, as yet unknown, aspects of people's experience. . . people who are living the experience are the experts—are the ones who really know how it is—what are the things that are difficult in this experience, what are the things that help, what are the things that made them increase their suffering or increase their well-being. . . they're the ones that know that—more than us—and that's the knowledge we want."

Initially, Dodds invited members of her groups to tell their story. She reports that, over time, after a number of sessions together, the richness of these stories increased. "People would give a fairly thin story at the beginning—as their trust in the group grew, their familarity and their ease, they would go

into their experiences in greater and greater depth—everybody else's experience and story would be triggers to help them think about their own and bring out the contradictions and similarities—just generally help them to go into it much deeper . . . and that was progressive, it went on—each meeting got deeper."

According to Dodds, as familiarity and trust grew among the participants, the meetings gradually became less dependent on her input as the participants spontaneously investigated, clarified, and identified common (and disparate) themes in their cancer experience.

METHOD

Dodds recorded group meetings and supplied participants with transcripts, thus giving them the opportunity to comment on their previous discussions. She also identified different themes in their conversations, which participants were invited to question or challenge. The endorsement of both the reports and the themes gave both the collection and preliminary analysis of the information significant credibility. "I'd done the first level of coding if you like—by dividing everthing up into paragraphs and giving headings . . . journalistic type headings. Seeing their story in a written, a pretty form . . . I made their own experiences somehow look special. There was a real validation, acknowledgment process. And, it increased their abilities to reflect—*all that* is a healing process."

By reflecting on commonalities and differences, the participants in Dodds's study were able to act in new ways towards their illness. With the support of other group participants, they were able to examine and reflect on the outcomes of their actions. "I guess what healing is for me and also became for most of the participants was, 'What areas of their life could they heal?' Several people joined the research process whose tumors shrank. . . so they talked about healing in their relationships, which promoted the healing of cancer; healing from working out role conflicts, which again had a direct impact on their physical health; healing through actually leaving a damaging relationship from which they saw direct consequences—a healing result in their physical bodies."

According to Dodds, therefore, the use of participatory action research in her practice was a way of combining inquiry and therapy. "The thing which really got me about this method was its dual research and therapeutic power—that in fact, it was a very strong therapeutic tool at the same time as you were collecting very rich data—because people could test the data at the same time as you were collecting it—like the example of a woman who died during the time that we were meeting. We were able to check if people's belief in meditation was dented by the fact that she had died anyway. Even though she was a really strong believer in meditation—and there she was, she died—so we really processed that and discussed it which of course meant that they grew from that experience instead of being left alone—so it was very much a combined practice with the research—the practice of facilitating healing."

REPRESENTATION

The opportunities for participants to create shared meanings in dialogue with each other promoted an alternative discourse about health and healing. When shared more widely, it meant that the research had even broader social implications. "It reminds me of the thing of throwing a stone into a lake—you know those rings—and the rings keep on going out wider and wider—and I continue to feel the presence of this research reverberating. . . . I can see how the more kind of this research that is done, it will change the construction of reality, the discourse—I know that my two research studies have helped validate, made more powerful, the idea of taking a proactive stance towards physical healing or mental healing through working on many other types of healing in one's life. Whether you are talking about a sick mind or a sick body, individuals can go beyond taking a pill or cutting it out or burning it—that there are definitely powerful things that people will do that will impact on their physical or mental health—very significant—this research process has helped draw that out and make it a reality instead of just a wish."

Dodds was, therefore, able to use action research in powerful ways to combine both research and practice to produce outcomes that were of immediate relevance to individual participants, but also had wider social implications.

3. Health Promotion and Community Development: Hazardous Waste Problems

Among the most powerful work health professionals can achieve is the willingness and ability to facilitate the research capabilities of citizen groups. Couto and Guthrie (1999) recount the efforts of community leaders to investigate issues related to hazardous waste dumping in their community. People in Bumpass Cove in Tennessee became aware of trucks dumping chemicals into landfill facilities in the area and formed the Bumpass Cove Citizens Group (BCCG) to halt these activities. After some initial success in having the state health department order a halt to the dumping of chemicals in the landfill, leaders of the group attended a workshop in which they learned how to track people who engaged in dumping, what they dumped, and health risks associated with chemicals.

Following the workshop, group leaders went to the state public health offices to research what had been dumped and were confronted with "pile after pile after pile" of papers, none of it in any particular order. They were able to use this information to create a booklet that enabled them to accurately identify hazardous wastes, their locations, and their sources. As one member of the group recalled:

> We were at this meeting and the big man at the health department was saying this [chemical] was not in these [the landfill] and that [chemical] was not in there and at last he said, 'How in the world would *you* know what was in there?' The health department had made it so confusing. We could go down there, and any file we asked for they could give to us, it could be in Greek and we wouldn't have known a thing about it. Now we spent all that time and effort at the Highlander Center and made that little booklet up. And we handed him the little booklet we made. It's showed all of the chemicals and the risks. And he said, 'Where did you get that?' If it hadn't been for the people at the Highland Center teaching us how to go about finding this information, we couldn't have known what to go down there and look for. (Couto & Guthrie, 1999, p. 116–117)

The group was thus empowered to take issue on a health concern of considerable importance to the health of the local community. As they acquired, distilled, and organized information (gathering and analyzing data), they acquired the capability to clarify and extend their understanding of the situation, not only regarding information related to toxicity and effects of chemicals but about the workings of the political and bureaucratic system that they eventually helped to make more effective. They became involved in a network of local organizations with similar concerns, extended their work to other issues, and helped form a statewide citizens coalition to deal with hazardous waste. As Couto notes:

> The outside assistance, publicity, and momentum of their group gave Bumpass Cove residents far more attention than they were accustomed to, and encourqaged some them, especially the women of the BCCG, to imagine a changed Bumpass Cove. Linda Walls, a BCCG leader, had modest but dramatically changed hopes for increased recreation, health care, cultural activities, and community bonds.(Couto & Guthrie,1999, p. 117)

They had hopes for a community center, like those they had seen in cities, and to continue focusing on their major concern—continuing to monitor the landfill and keeping people healthy. They also gained greater insight into the politics of their situation and the limits of their power, a mixed blessing that brought some sadness. As one of the group noted:

> We wised up. In some ways that was really good and some ways that was really sad. . . We lost the innocence that we had of just living here and feeling like the government was protecting us. . . We learned not to trust, and that's a shame—not to trust the health department, not to trust the government, to learn to trust yourself and check things out. . . . To question, that's what we've learned." (Couto & Guthrie, 1999, p. 118)

In Chapter 1, we noted the possibility of developmental action research processes that can move a group from a specific, local issue into broader and broader arenas of activity. It is not only the *scope* of the work that indicates its developmental nature, but also the impact it has on people. As they develop their capacities to understand and influence issues affecting their lives, they become stronger and wiser in the process and assist the broader community to understand and develop the capacity to deal with the issues at hand.

4. Creative Prevention Strategies: Hospitals and the Community

Kretzman and McKnight (1993) present a model of community building that demonstrates how innovative hospitals are demonstrating a new understanding of their roles by stressing a variety of creative prevention strategies that support and nurture the health of people in the communities they serve. They suggest that by rediscovering hospitals as assets within the community, hospitals may use their resources to catalyze developments that diminish the need for provision of very expensive care—care that may become futile in the face of growing health problems in poorer communities.

Their process for using hospitals as resources for prevention programs, services, and activities requires an initial investment in action research processes to:

- Review the assets of the hospital—personnel, space and facilities, materials and equipment, expertise, economic power
- Map community assets as potential partners for local hospitals—community associations and organizations; public institutions such as schools, police, parks services, and so on; local businesses; special interest groups—youth, seniors, and so on
- Build productive and mutually beneficial relationships between hospitals and community partners

They describe a number of these types of activities in which hospitals in the United States have engaged:

- A hospital forms a partnership with an alternative high school, the local police department, and a social service agency in order to provide programs that prevent the institutionalization of troubled youth.
- A hospital works with a local health clinic to provide special services that are more culturally sensitive to the needs of the neighborhood's Asian population.

- A hospital forms a network of community barbershops and churches to conduct blood pressure screenings for young men in the neighborhood.
- A local hospital sponsors a Chinese health fair in which local volunteers provide translations of relevant information, doctors donate prizes, and students from a local school perform.
- A hospital develops a community sex education program for fourth through eighth graders at seven local schools. One of these schools has 500 students enrolled in the program and has seen a dramatic reduction in pregnancies.
- A hospital develops a partnership with the local police department to get referrals for its rape counseling program and its child abuse clinic.
- A hospital forms a partnership with a large manufacturing company and an association of community residents to rehabilitate existing housing in the neighborhood.
- A hospital forms a partnership with a chain of department stores to open neighborhood health clinics in two of its branches.
- A hospital develops relationships with local factories and businesses to provide referrals for a substance abuse recovery program.
- People who are enrolled in a hospital's methadone program initiate an AIDS volunteer organization in which volunteers from the neighborhood provide companionship, run errands, pay bills, and intercede with landlords on behalf of people with AIDS.

In each case, the extent to which local people have assisted in the research required for instigating these activities was varied. Success of the initiatives, however, rested on the extent to which hospitals were able to build bridges between themselves and community resources. Initial investigations, envisaged as action research processes, provide the means not only to develop the required relationships, but also to determine the resources available, the needs to be met, and the processes for meeting those needs.

5. Primary Health Care: Investigating Alcohol Issues

A central focus of both comprehensive primary health care and health promotion continues the contextual determinants of health, including environmental factors and patterned social behaviors within any social context. One of the authors of this text (Genat) has almost 20 years experience using action research a vehicle for community development in health. The example that follows emerged from work in a small rural town.

INTRODUCTION

I received a call from the manager of an Indigenous Health Service (I.H.S.) in a small town who asked me to work on problems associated with alcohol in the local indigenous community. My first task was to facilitate a meeting of I.H.S. workers and people from within the community who had an interest in alcohol issues.

From the beginning, the project became a shared inquiry—an action research project. Initially, I asked the participants what they wanted to know about alcohol. Questions such as "Why do people drink?" and "What's bad about drinking?" were answered by seeking accounts of participants' experiences of alcohol use in the community. Other questions, such as "What's the problem?" "What can we do if it's up to people themselves?" "What do other people think?" and "What can the I.H.S. do about it?" gave participants the idea to develop a small project that involved consulting community members and seeking responses from a sample of households.

ENTRY INTO THE RESEARCH SITE

Participants in the group soon realized that such a project faced some serious problems. They expressed concern that such a project in a small community, where the use of alcohol was a commonplace social activity, meant that they were likely to face either hostility or ridicule from people consuming alcohol at home. They decided that entering a household where people were drinking would require considerable forethought. How were they to legitimate "poking their nose" into other peoples' affairs? How could they justify their interest? I suggested we use role-plays

and socio-drama to explore and rehearse approaches to their task.

Participants rehearsed a variety of scenarios and the roles I.H.S. workers and their colleagues could adopt to legitimate entry into households and undertake their inquiries in an acceptable manner. Eventually, the group decided that as I.H.S. workers they could legitimately investigate the pain and suffering related to alcohol use experienced by their clients. On this basis, the health workers visited households in the community asking the question "What pain and suffering does alcohol cause your family?"

ACTION PLANNING

The pain and suffering related to alcohol identified by the I.H.S. workers in their inquiries within the community included:

- Personal illness and injury
- Kids being neglected by parents and placed in the care of others
- Old people missing meals and baths and becoming sick
- Families experiencing poverty due to consistent heavy fines from overzealous policing

While each of the findings emerged from at least two households, the last finding was found in every household visited. Further research revealed that in eight months, indigenous people in a community of 250 had paid $197,471 in fines, mostly related to alcohol offenses (ALS, 1994).

The action planning session that comprised the Think component of the Look-Think-Act cycle included the problem solving matrix of Figure 8.1

Subsequently, participants in the project decided which problems had most *priority*, identified the *causes* of these problems, linked the causes to possible *strategies,* and identified *actions* required to engage these strategies. These strategies, undertaken by indigenous participants and their agencies, helped to improve policing and change the policing culture. In conjunction with harm minimization strategies that were also adopted, the health status of the community improved markedly.

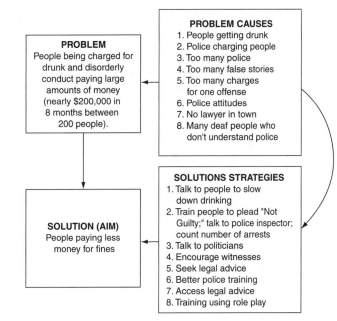

Figure 8.1
Problem Solving Matrix

6. *Parent Participation and Involvement in the Care of a Hospitalized Child*

The account that follows provides an example of a program that, though participatory, has not been developed as an action research process. The lack of clarity of the role, duties, and/or activities of the participants suggests how a systematic process of exploration and analysis might have provided the basis for more effective participation by parents.

Darbyshire (1994) recounts the experiences of a group of parents who either lived with or spent most of the day with their child in a Scottish pediatric hospital, participating with nurses in the care of their children. Levels of participation and involvement of parents varied, some carrying out activities related to basic mothering, while others were able to attain levels of autonomy and expertise that enabled them to apply technical care at a level implying a deeper sense of being an integral and essential part of their child's hospital experience. Though others may have had a general desire to help care for their child, they lacked sufficient knowledge of the child's condition to allow them confidently to take a more active role.

A study of this situation revealed that parents who lived in the hospital with their children appeared to have no clear understanding of the nature or extent of what their participation might be. It did not appear to be an arrangement that was openly negotiated, and there was considerable uncertainty among parents about their roles. In these circumstances, parents often found the process of participating in the care of their child fraught with tensions—they were uncertain and confused about what they were allowed or expected to do. Parents took their cues from other resident parents and, especially in situations where the child was severely ill, tended to participate less directly, the technical tasks or physical procedures carried out by nurses being elevated in importance.

Darbyshire noted that "Parents participated more when they were asked informally and unthreateningly by nurses whether they might like to help with a particular aspect of their child's care. This encouragement also extended to the performance of more technical tasks ... although parents tended to be taught more formally how to carry out these procedures, rather than gently encouraged" (1994, p. 190–191). Parents appeared particularly appreciative of nurses who al-

lowed them to make choices about the extent and degree of their participation. Although some parents carried out aspects of their child's care on their own initiative, the control of parent participation rested principally with the nursing staff. Parents played with their children, and "kept vigil" in order to minimize the trauma of hospitalization.

The nurses perspectives on the readiness of parents to participate in the care of their child was based on assessments of a parent's willingness, interest, timing, ability, and the nature of the tasks in which they might become involved. This type of assessment was largely intuitive and not part of a well-articulated set of practices. Despite this, nurses often claimed "that it was valuable to have close contact with parents because they were the experts, the people who knew their child best" (Darbyshire, 1994, p. 202).

Parent participation in the care of their child, therefore, seemed to largely rest upon a set of unspoken agreements that were rarely discussed formally. The creation, control, and determination of parent participation was generally up to the nurses, according to their own determinations of what was possible, and what each parent was capable of achieving. Parent participation was largely dependant, therefore, on the development of relationships with ward staff, rather than the clear explication of a set of procedures or guidelines.

Nurses in the study described an "inform and leave" strategy in which they provided parents with information and encouragement to participate, then left them to decide whether or not they wished to do so. Some nurses also described how they tried to promote participation by encouraging parents to feel free to do whatever they did for the child at home. Exclusionary practices adopted in relation to access to use of hospital facilities, like the kitchen, created an unrecognized tension in this regard.

What seemed missing from the nurses' and parents' accounts was any real sense of involvement, reciprocity, or mutuality. Impressions gained from participant accounts indicated that parents functioned as helpers, a role akin to that of an unqualified member of ward staff. Darbyshire suggests that this state of affairs might have resulted from the impact it had on the nurses' sense of professional identity:

Nurses described a tension wherein they recognized the importance of allowing and encouraging parents to undertake more of their child's care, but also recognized that this could seem diminishing to their sense of self as nurses. For some nurses, sharing care with and involving parents was not a calling forth of greater connectedness with a whole family. Rather, it seemed that by "handing over" aspects of care that had traditionally been viewed as their's, nurses then saw nothing of comparable value with which replace them. There was a tension apparent here whereby some nurses felt that by encouraging parents to undertake more of their child's care, they as nurses, were consequently diminished (Darbyshire, 1994, p. 208)

7. *Change Management in an Interdisciplinary Inpatient Facility within Health Services*

INTRODUCTION

Barker and Barker (1994) report on the use of action research for organizational change within an interdisciplinary inpatient unit. Applied to organizational change, they describe a six-phase action research model:

1. **Diagnosis:** The initial phase involves preliminary assessment of issues facing the organization using observation, documentation, or interviews. From this initial diagnosis, objectives and direction for the change effort are developed.
2. **Data Gathering:** During this phase, additional information is gathered from various groups/individuals to further identify specific patterns of strengths and weaknesses in task accomplishment and interpersonal relations.
3. **Feedback to the Client Group:** The designated change agent, having categorized the collected data, then shares the information with the client group. This information is provided to inform the client group about the state of the organization and encourages their involvement in the change process.
4. **Data Discussion and Plans for Adjustment:** The client group reacts to the information and action plans are developed.
5. **Action:** During the action phase, the client group implements the plans.
6. **Evaluation:** Information is gathered to determine if designated changes have begun, become accepted, or if further adjustment is needed. Continuous cycles of the action research cycle provide monitoring and management processes.

AN ORGANIZATIONAL CHANGE PROCESS

Barker and Barker describe an organizational change process instigated by the new director of a well-established substance abuse inpatient unit in a large university teaching hospital.

Entry

The authors highlight the challenge of working with professionals from a variety of disciplines. The new di-

rector in the unit, a mental health professional, established a management team that met weekly, initially to identify issues and outstanding concerns. The concerns of all staff, psychosocial and nursing staff, and physicians were presented at meetings.

Diagnosis

Initially, key informants from the three staff groups represented on the management team were interviewed. Existing policy documents and procedures also were reviewed. Specific objectives were identified from these initial inquiries:

1. Address initial staff issues of interdisciplinary conflict, low morale, and high turnover
2. Determine perceptions of the needs of the unit
3. Identify target areas for change
4. Develop change interventions involving staff members
5. Implement change interventions
6. Evaluate change interventions
7. Provide for continuing the change process (steps 1–6)

Data Collection and Analysis (Data Discussion)

The management team and key personnel from each staff group developed a needs assessment instrument to provide staff with the means to rate staff relations, program components, unit leadership, and policies and procedures. The survey also included some more open-ended questions on staff perceptions. Of the 30 instruments distributed, 21 were completed.

Staff received the results verbally at staff meetings and as a written report. Ninety-five percent of respondents identified a staff-related issue as one of the top two priorities of the unit and 61% of these regarded interdisciplinary issues, including the needs for trust, cooperation, respect, open communication, teamwork, and team building.

Planning

Planning is required at all points of the change process. All stakeholders need to clearly define the way changes in their practices will contribute to program needs.

To continue to involve staff members in the change efforts, multidisciplinary committees were formed to develop interventions to address major programmatic needs identified. An initial staff meeting was held from which staff members volunteered to serve on committees of interest to them. An education committee composed of nursing and psychosocial staff was formed to review the existing educational program and treatment schedule. Another committee was formed to develop an inservice schedule based on unit needs, and still another was formed to focus on the point system used to reward patients for treatment progress. The management team agreed to focus on developing written policies and procedures to guide unit staff. (Barker & Barker, 1994, p. 8)

Action

Each committee developed draft proposals on policies and procedures, which they circulated to other staff inviting both comment and participation.

The education committee developed an integrated educational program appropriate for patients in early withdrawal. The inservice committee developed a monthly inservice schedule and arranged for appropriate presenters, and the point system committee revised the criteria and procedures for monitoring patient progress in treatment. The management group provided written policies addressing major issues, such as smoking on the unit, shutting down the unit when contraband was found, telephone and television use, developing agendas for morning report (rounds) and treatment team meetings, and passes to leave the unit. A series of six basic communication sessions focusing on help-

ing skills (active listening, effective feedback) were also developed and provided for nursing staff members' professional development. (Barker & Barker, 1994, p.8)

Review

Twelve months after the initial needs assessment, the action research process was formally reviewed across the unit, and new goals were established for the next 12 months.

IMPLICATIONS OF THE STUDY

Barker and Barker (1994) identify some particular implications in the use of action research for mental health administrators from their study. They suggest that action research provides:

- A systematic way of managing change within interdisciplinary contexts that encompasses needs assessment, planning, implementation, and evaluation
- An organizational climate of collaboration that supports participatory management, team building, and relationships of trust
- Opportunities for staff ownership and acceptance of change processes
- Mechanisms for management–staff communication that also support quality improvement processes
- Mechanisms to demonstrate accountability through empirical data on policy and program implementation

8. Incorporating the Social Context: Collaborative Reflection within a Family Practice

INTRODUCTION

Meg Bond (1999) reports on a professional development project directed towards enhancing the knowledge and practices of health professionals working in contexts where poverty was a significant feature of the situation. The intent was to "enable workers to develop empowering rather than victim-blaming or dependency-inducing intervention strategies" (Bond, 1999, p. 3). The participants were a general practitioner (family physician) and the nine nursing and administrative staff members working within his practice.

ENTRY

In order for researchers to engage with the staff in the practice, they negotiated joint roles with the staff acting as co-researchers. A division of labor emerged where both staff members and researchers undertook specific tasks with a clear intent to relieve staff, where possible, of any extra imposition on their existing work. The researchers, for instance, undertook the bulk of the writing.

METHOD

Members of the project staff and the primary health care team met in two-week intervals, sharing and recording their experiences, issues, and perspectives on poverty. In addition, the primary health care team members began to collect data on poverty in their local area and engage with staff in related agencies. Several focus groups emerged from these networks and served as a basis for even broader participation.

DATA COLLECTION AND ANALYSIS— PARTICIPANT PERSPECTIVES

Participants reported improved relationships and teamwork, higher self-esteem, and clearer role definition. Bond (1999) also reports shifts in participant attitudes towards poverty, a greater understanding of poverty, particularly within the local area, and more insight into the links between poverty and health. Subsequently, participants developed a community profile of poverty for use by both themselves and staff in other agencies. This profile provided health professionals with a contextual understanding of the poverty and suffering of their clients. Greater interagency collaboration also emerged from the project.

DATA COLLECTION AND ANALYSIS— RESEARCHER PERSPECTIVES

Bond suggests that "four interactive team learning processes that revolve around collective thinking and action were identifiable . . . framing/reframing, experimenting, crossing boundaries and integrating perspectives explain the processes of converting 'fragmented' individual learning into 'pooled' then 'synergistic' and finally 'continuous' team learning." (Bond, 1999, p.12)

In conclusion, Bond suggests, "adoption of an action research strategy ensured a combination of disciplined inquiry, ownership of change initiatives, evaluation of the project, and dissemination of the findings . . . participants enhanced their understandings of the health implications of structural factors, including income distribution and unemployment, and took steps to enable poor families . . . to maximize their entitlements to welfare benefits." (Bond, 1999, p.15)

9. *Developing Acute Care Protocols in Accident and Emergency*

McElroy and Shepherd (1999) report on an action research project investigating procedures for the assessment and management of self-harming patients of an Accident and Emergency clinic in a general hospital. The project team included two researchers in collaboration with two nurses from the A & E clinic.

Entry

By working collaboratively with two health professionals stationed within the unit, the researchers were able to engage the interest of 90% of the A & E staff.

Framing

The researchers presented four vignettes of critical incidents to all A & E staff and conducted interviews concerning their responses.

Data Collection and Analysis

Staff received transcribed records of their interviews along with a thematic analysis of their content. The researchers encouraged them to question the categories of analysis and contribute their own themes.

Action

In response to the analysis, participants conducted trials of a number of risk assessment tools. They also developed a risk assessment tool for implementation by the nurses involved at first point of contact with clients. A self-harm planning team was also established to maintain ongoing monitoring of the strategy.

10. *Integrating the Isolated Aged into Community Practice*

INTRODUCTION

Moyer, Coristine, Jamault, Roberge, and O'Hagan (1999) employed action research methods to gain access, assess needs, and design interventions to integrate older people at risk of losing their independence into the community. The researchers conducted the Canadian study in an urban, French-speaking community with a high number of residents over 65-years-old, living alone, and having a household income under the poverty line. Of 100 clients contacted in the first year, 37 emerged as participants. They received an average of five visits between their first contact and the end of the second year.

ENTRY

The public health nurses conducting the study initially gained entry to the community through the development of an inventory of services for the aged in collaboration with local agencies. By accompanying agency workers on outreach visits and hosting a church supper, the researchers gained client contacts. Initially they telephoned clients, then followed up with a home visit. The nurse researchers attempted to establish friendliness and warmth in their relationships with the clients, conversed in the client's language of choice, and negotiated consent and a verbal contract concerning participation. "The contract had four components: exploring issues related to independent living; mutual goal setting and development of an action plan; scheduling of visits; and agreement to reassess at three monthly intervals" (Moyer et al., 1999, p. 106).

DATA COLLECTION

Field notes, case records, interviews, records of meetings, and project briefings constituted the major sources of data within the study. The researchers assessed the functional capacity of participants using established research instruments. Observations and informal conversations enabled researchers to analyze the extent of participants' social networks and supports.

DATA ANALYSIS

Transcripts of interviews were analyzed using NUD-IST. The researchers built a picture of the participants' social networks and interactions in relation to daily living activities and analyzed their extent using an "ecomap." With each client, they developed a set of goals to support their independence and a related action plan to assess during return visits. The ongoing action-reflection cycle with each of the participants—data collection and analysis—provided data of considerable depth through the life of the study. Using this data, researchers developed a profile of "older people in need" by comparing the data of clients with one another and clients with non-clients.

FINDINGS

Moyer and her colleagues suggest that in order to gain in-depth data about isolated clients, usual methods of surveying by telephone, brief observation, or other rapid screening methods are insufficient. In order to gather salient data, they suggest, home visits are required by a practitioner/investigator both skilled and knowledgeable in the field (in this case, aged care) and operating within a holistic framework. They also highlight the significance of forming and maintaining in-depth relationships with the participants over a period of time.

The study concludes that:

> Primary prevention requires a population-based approach to help older people to age in a healthy way through raising awareness and educating the public about the importance of social networks and by using community development approaches to strengthen support networks in the community. (Moyer et al., 1999, p. 110)

11. Developing Clinical Protocols for Cataract Surgery

Rose, Waterman, Mcleod, and Tullo (1999) report on the use of action research in parallel with a randomized control trial comparing two management protocols governing the organization and implementation of day surgery for cataract.

THE SETTING

There were two sites involved in the investigation of the two protocols: a peripheral clinic located within a district general hospital and a specialist eye hospital. The management protocols governing day surgery for cataract are outlined in Table 8.1

In order to implement the study, a qualified opthalmic nurse was recruited to the peripheral clinic to provide immediate pre-operative assessments for the experimental group and post-operative care. A nursing auxiliary, two nurses and a doctor, undertook pre-operative assessments in the eye hospital and doctors and optometrists provided post-operative care.

INTEGRATING RESEARCH OF CLINICAL PRACTICE USING ACTION RESEARCH

In conducting the research, the researchers acknowledge that, in the real world, it is impossible to control variables affecting practice. Therefore, prior to the im-plementation of the randomized control trial, action research was undertaken with the participation of clinic staff, researchers, and grant holders to investigate how to integrate the trial into the running of the clinic.

> A series of meetings to which all interested parties were invited was held. At these meetings, issues such as the continuing education of staff, the logistics of explaining the study to patients, randomization, ensuring the patients were ushered to the correct member of staff at the correct time, and ensuring that those coming by hospital transport did not get missed because they were not following the usual pattern of clinic attendance, were discussed. (Rose et al., 1999, p. 1517)

Rose et al. report that the action research process ensured that they addressed all stakeholder issues and concerns prior to the trial. When procedural issues arose during implementation, an ongoing participatory forum existed as a means to generate solutions and contribute to "a working culture of evidence-based practice." The authors conclude that "Although the basic study design was a randomized control trial, setting up the trial within an action research framework enabled a flexible handling of events as they arose without disastrous consequences for the setting or the study" (Rose et al., 1999, p. 1518).

Table 8.1

Management Models of Patients Undergoing Day-Case Cataract Surgery

	Experimental Group	Control Group
Step 1	Referral by GP	
Step 2	Peripheral Clinic: Cataract Confirmed	Peripheral Clinic: Cataract Confirmed
Step 3	Preoperatively assessed by ophthalmic nurse (or optometrist)	Diary booked for pre-op assessment at eye hospital
		Pre-Op assessment 2–4 weeks prior to surgery
Step 4	Surgery at Main Hospital	Surgery at Main Hospital
Step 5	Post-op visits to peripheral clinic—seen by ophthalmic nurse, doctor and optometrist	Post-op visits to peripheral clinic—seen by doctor and optometrist

(Rose et al. 1999: p. 1516)

12. Action Research and Evidence-Based Wound Management

INTRODUCTION

Selim, Bashford, and Grossman (2001) report on a participatory action research project into effective wound management in a community nursing organization. A participatory action research group searched for evidence to support the organization's wound-cleansing policy that advocated cleansing a leg ulcer using either tap water in a bowl or shower (clean technique) or using a dressing pack and sterile saline (aseptic technique). An item in an internal newsletter and announcements at regular monthly staff meetings were the means for the recruitment of participants from among the community nurses within the organization.

FRAMING THE STUDY

The first meeting of the participatory action research group resolved to examine evidence-based practice and leg ulcers. By the fourth meeting, it had narrowed the topic to the issue of tap water cleansing for chronic leg ulcers. The question driving the group was: "Is this acceptable practice for community nurses?" (Selim et al., 2001, p. 374).

Members of the PAR group also read and shared articles of interest, and these initial inquiries formed a knowledge base to guide decision-making in the development of an action plan. On the basis of initial research into wound management techniques, the PAR group concluded that either warm tap water or warm saline are acceptable cleansing solutions.

DATA COLLECTION AND ANALYSIS

The PAR group surveyed other nursing staff and received a 71% response to their questionnaire concerning the preferred wound cleansing methods. Initially, over 70% of nurses indicated that they used dressing packs and saline rather than tap water. Explanations included concerns about infection using the tap water technique; unsanitary conditions; lack of access to running water, a towel, and a bucket; and habit.

ACTION

The PAR group concluded that concerns about infection were the major reason nurses would not use the clean technique and disseminated articles about wound cleansing with tap water and the importance of hand washing.

EVALUATION

A further survey in 1999 indicated there had been a 21% increase in the use of the clean technique subsequent to the actions of the PAR group.

13. Collaborative Inquiry into a WHO Protocol: Stories of Family Physicians

Mash and Meulenberg-Buskens (2001) report on a collaborative inquiry/action research project conducted by a group of general practitioners (family physicians) aimed at adapting the World Health Organizan's (WHO) educational program Mental Disorders in Primary Care for South African GPs.

ESTABLISHMENT

Invitations to join the collaborative inquiry group (CIG) were spread through word of mouth and also advertised through the South African Academy of Family Practice and Primary Care. After an introductory meeting, a diverse group of 10 participants from both private and public practices located in suburban, inner city, rural areas, and townships committed themselves to the project for six months.

DESIGN

The CIG undertook four cycles of action-reflection—each lasting from four to six weeks. Individual participants incorporated structured exercises into their work to enhance their own reflexivity in relation to their individual implementation of the educational package.

DATA COLLECTION AND ANALYSIS

The major focus of the group meetings was the WHO educational program and its adaption to the context of the physicians' work. Group meetings including experiences, perspectives, and reflections on practice were recorded on audiotape. Group facilitators also recorded notes on emerging themes. A written summary documented important decisions and discussions and was distributed to participants.

Participants also recorded observations and narrative accounts of implementing the educational package within their own clinic. Training within the sessions and a set of structured exercises strengthened their capacity to engage in an unfamiliar practice; in particular, the extent of disclosure required and its emotional components. The researchers suggest that in order to practice and observe practice at the same time, the participants needed to imagine a researcher who sat on their shoulder without judgment,

observing while they practiced, noting issues and events that sparked interest and ongoing reactions. This capacity the researchers termed an ability to "hold it lightly."

Participants communicated reflections electronically and an archive developed on the list-server used for the purpose. At the end of the six-month period, each participant wrote a personal reflection about his or her inquiry processes. These were also shared electronically on the list server. The first author analyzed the data on the list server and wrote a summary of emerging themes. Participants debated this anlaysis and the emergent themes in the final collaborative session aimed at developing a degree of consensus.

Because the inquiry focused on the implementation of the WHO guidelines and demanded reflection based on experience, some difficulties emerged:

> One problem was that we were used to asserting our conclusions in the group without showing how we arrived at them. Group members had to learn to document what happened in a brief narrative form so they could show how they arrived at their personal reflection and learning. We developed the concept of a portfolio of personal stories, rather like a collection of paintings. After this, the process of reflection on the portfolio could also be recorded and any new concepts or theories summarized. The act of writing was found to be not just a way of recording our thoughts, but in itself a way of thinking and reflecting. (Mash & Meulenberg-Buskens, 2001, p. 1113)

OUTCOMES

The researchers reported a "creative tension" within the CIG process as each participant was engaged in their own personal learning journey as well as the collaborative learning journey of the group. Nevertheless, they suggest that for the participants both processes enriched each other. Some resistance emerged among the participants, most who were initially unfamiliar with the degree of self-reflection required by the method. Nevertheless, the researchers indicate that participants remained committed and experienced significant learning. They conclude that CIG is a useful method when health professionals wish to reflect upon and change their practice.

14. The Oncology Clinic Tea Trolley: Community Development in Health

Menon (1993) describes an action research project she undertook in her role as the health promotion officer in a large tertiary hospital.

FRAMING THE PROJECT

In the early days of her employment as the health promotion officer in the hospital, Menon became aware, from her informal conversations with people, of the need to better support cancer patients. She inquired into the issue using informal interviews (hallway conversations) and a small survey with patients, nurses, and relatives seeking their experiences and perceptions of cancer treatment and care. The data revealed:

> "The lack of a caring human face" and "the lack of a person to look after me." Without exception, all patients and relatives identified other patients and relatives, rather than doctors and nurses, as the most beneficial and important source for gaining meaningful information and caring support—"The only person who really understands what it is like is someone who has cancer has been through it all. (Menon, 1993, p. 68)

ENGAGING THE PARTICIPANTS

Menon identified the need for cancer patients to talk about diagnosis and treatment and to receive greater support while they waited for treatment. She recognized the potential of a tea trolley service to catalyze a support group among the patients and relatives who often sat silently in uncomfortable chairs for several hours in a depressing waiting room. She reports that the tea trolley gradually became a familiar part of the routine of the waiting room and her offers of tea became the catalyst for friendly conversations.

CYCLES WITHIN CYCLES OF ACTION AND REFLECTION

Further data gathering and analysis emerged spontaneously around the tea trolley. Concerns that were expressed by one patient became shared issues to be further investigated by the waiting room group. Experiences of other patients, the knowledge of the nurses and doctors, and pamphlets, newspapers, and books became further sources of information. Patients and waiting relatives identified emerging themes—care, support, and treatment—and initiated new actions—swapping diets and recipes, exchanging ideas, and discussing the effects of various intervention strategies. Further action and reflection occurred as patients engaged in role-plays of potential interactions with doctors or used trial and error to rehearse questions they wished to ask.

OUTCOME

These activities captured the interest and support of patients, relatives, and other hospital staff. Gradually, Menon herself became only an adjunct to the service as the patients and their relatives became involved in running the tea trolley service and extending the support network beyond the hospital into the community.

15. Entry to Cross-Cultural Inquiry: The House Party

Wong (1993) shares her experience working with women of the Kampuchean community in order to assist them to gain better access to community health services.

BACKGROUND

Wong initially worked with the Federation of Family Planning Associations in Malaysia and reports how she "encountered" the House Party strategy of health promotion during visits to Malaysian towns with a field worker:

> [The field worker's] first initiative was to discover a person willing to host a small gathering of friends and neighbors in her own house. In this "tea party" atmosphere, she talked to the guests about their everyday lives in terms of the expectations and responsibilities for the life of the family. . . . Muslim culture and custom forbids the use of contraception, but the relaxed atmosphere of the House Party made it possible for the Malaysian women to share experiences and to acknowledge each others difficulties. . . . It seemed to me that as a social arrangement, the House Party had none of the threatening overtones associated with more formal learning contexts and might be a key to reaching isolated communities. (Wong, 1993, p. 41)

Later, Wong worked as an outreach worker for a community health service in an urban context where refugees and immigrants were housed in high-rise, inner city housing apartments. She observed that residents in such situations became very isolated, an unfortunate situation for groups whose lives and social support networks had suffered disruption through migration. She suggests:

> For these reasons the process of "access and linking" needs to utilize the mutual support inherent in their natural environment and natural networks. The House Party processes can effectively link workers to the targeted community, the community to the worker, community members to each other, and the community to specific projects. (Wong, 1993, p. 42)

ENTRY

In order to set up the House Party, Wong describes how she established relationships with people by "hanging around" housing estates or making links through an existing client of the community health service. Once the health worker has established a level of trust in her relationship, the client was informed about the intended purpose and content of a House Party session and encouraged to gather people together from her network of friends and acquaintances.

INQUIRY

Wong provides the example of a young sole parent from the Kampuchean community. The woman was diagnosed with a mental illness by another health professional, but Wong was convinced she was suffering the effects of social dislocation and post-war trauma. In her despair, the Kampuchean woman had discarded religious artifacts and amulets associated with her faith. Wong felt the cure for her condition lay in the healing networks of her own community. "Sadly, what K had unwittingly relinquished, when she disposed of the ritual objects of her faith, was the spiritual connection with her upbringing—the basis of her confidence that she was a fit person to care for her own children" (Wong, 1993, p. 45).

COLLABORATIVE INQUIRY

Wong reports that when K moved to a new dwelling, the House Party provided opportunities for interaction, sharing, and healing:

> When K finally moved out of her flat—leaving the evil spirits behind her—we exploited the Buddhist custom of blessing a new dwelling and held a House Party to coincide with the first birthday of her baby daughter. . . the House Party amounted to a healing ceremony validated through the participation of members of K's own community, including her own children. (Wong, 1993, p. 46)

Wong's account reveals that the House Party process enables the development of trusting relationships without threatening overtones. Within this informal, mutually supportive context, the practitioner/ researcher is able to inquire into the experience of isolated groups, identify shared themes, and enable community action to establish healthy and supportive environments.

OUTCOME

In her conclusion, Wong suggests:

> Listening to these women led me to the realization. . . that what counts is a person's sensitivity to the wishes and experience of her clients. . . I also need to be flexible enough to be comfortable with the issues as defined by the people themselves. (Wong, 1993, p. 47)

On-Line Resources

Introduction

In the past few years, on-line resources to support action research in health have proliferated. A reasonably superficial search will uncover a vast array of links that provide health practitioners with access to resources specifically relevant to their work. By judicious selection, action researchers may link to the courses, project descriptions, organizations, resources, listserves, and/or papers most suited to their purposes.

On-Line Web Searches

Web searches may be conducted to acquire understanding of action research processes, to acquire data relevant to a particular topic or issue, or to extend a literature review. A broad search may be made using any of the standard search engines like Yahoo, Altavista, and so on.

To conduct an on-line web search, researchers should:

- **Carefully define the topic:** A succinct definition of a topic aids clarity and precision. It ensures you get the type of information you require. A description that is too general or lengthy will not give sufficient focus to the search.
- **Identify key terms:** Key terms identify the type of information required. Select two or three terms that define the nature of the topic. If you were searching for information about the development of care plans, you might use the terms "health," "care," "plans."
- **Log on to search function:** Log on to a search engine (by clicking on to the "search" icon, then selecting the desired search engine).
- **Enter key terms:** Enter previously identified key terms.
- **Refine the search:** Often an initial search will not provide appropriate sources. It may identify many sources only peripherally related to the topic investigated, or

fail to identify an adequate body of resources. The search may be refined by changing the key terms, or by adding another term that locates the topic more precisely (e.g., the terms "community," "health," and "care" may be substituted for the previous key terms). It might also be possible to refine the search by identifying the years to be searched or the type of publication to be included in the search.

- **Evaluating sources:** Web searches may identify a large array of material, some of which is of questionable value. Researchers should evaluate the quality of material to ensure its adequacy or appropriateness to the study in which they are involved.

Useful Websites

The following list provides but a small sample of websites giving information about action research. There are some limitations to these materials, insofar as even new sites go temporarily off-line, and some become superseded. In some instances, those authoring the sites have no resources to update the information and they become outdated. Those limitations aside, however, there is a wide range of resources having the potential to greatly enrich an action research project by providing links with practitioners with similar professional or health interests.

The following categories differentiate between types of sites, but these are not mutually exclusive—some sites are linked to others or link to similar sources. A brief search, however, will provide researchers with an understanding of the range of sites relevant to their purposes and contexts. A rather simple, but effective, method of identifying action research sites is to enter "Action Research Health" as descriptors in a search engine and review the sites presented. More focused searches using more specific descriptors will reveal sites with more relevant information.

General Website Resources

These websites are multi-dimensional sites, each providing access or links to a broad range of topics and resources related to action research. They include literature, links, classes, resources, papers, publications, and descriptions of projects.

Action Research

Literature and websites. A checklist for action research. A definition of action research.

http:/ /www.ched.coventry.ac.uk/Taskforce/actionre.htm

Action Research at Queen's University

Provides excellent links to programs, conferences, sites, resources, publications, and student and faculty reports related to action research.

http:/ /educ.queensu.ca/~ar

Action Research Resources

University of Minnesota

http:/ /www.extension.umn.edu/~hoefer/educdsgn/actresrc.htm

Action Research Resources

An excellent list of links to many good action research sites.

http:/ /www.trinityvt.edu/edsite/action.htm

/NRM_changelinks/action research resources

List links to many useful action research websites.

http:/ /nrm.massey.ac.nz/changelinks/ar.html

Action Research Guidelines and Methodology

These sites provide specific guidance to those wishing to extend their knowledge of and skills in action research methods.

A Beginner's Guide to Action Research

A very useful and comprehensive guide to action from Bob Dick.

http:/ /ousd.k12.ca.us/netday/links/Action_Research/begin_guide_action_research

Action Research Methodology

An overview of the methodological approach of action research.

http:/ /www.web.net/~robrien/papers/arfinal.html

Women's Health

The Women's Health and Action Research Centre (WHARC) is a registered, non-profit organization committed to the promotion of women's reproductive health in sub-Saharan Africa. The Center's primary mission is to conduct multi-disciplinary and collaborative research, advocacy, and training on issues relating to the reproductive health of women.

http:/ /www.hsph.harvard.edu/ajrh/wharc.htm

The Feminist.com site includes health and sexuality resources.

http:/ /www.feminist.com/about/

The British Columbia Centre for Excellence for Women's Health provides information about resources, publications, and grants related to women's health.

http://www.bccewh.bc.ca/

The site of the Office of Women's Health, the U.S. Government agency promoting research, information, and service to women's health

http://www.4woman.gov/owh/

Community Organizations

The Public Citizen Health Research Group is a national (U.S.) non-profit public interest organization that provides information on a wide range of health issues. The Health Research Group promotes research-based, system-wide changes in health care policy and provides oversight concerning drugs, medical devices, doctors and hospitals, and occupational health.

http://www.citizen.org/hrg/

The Poverty & Race Research Action Council is a non-partisan, national, not-for-profit organization convened by major civil rights, civil liberties, and anti-poverty groups. Its purpose is to link social science research to advocacy work to address problems at the intersection of race and poverty. The site incorporates health-related links—health; diet and nutrition; women, families, and children—and provides information on relevant articles, literature, and grants.

http://www.prrac.org/

The Action Research Health Care Network presents ways that action research can be used for health care exploration and change.

http://www.triangle.co.uk/ear/pdf/05–2-rn.pdf

Social Action for Health is a community-based organization that has the aim of facilitating solution-focused changes in practice that lead to increased equity and health gain for local people.

http://www.safh.org.uk/about/index.htm

Commercial/Community Websites offering health information and advice to the public.

http://www.healthandage.com/ (Health and age)

http://www.webmd.com/ (General)

Government-Sponsored Sites

Health Canada is a government-sponsored site providing research information in support of decision-making in the management of the Canadian health system. It provides links to the Canadian Institute of Health Research, the Health Transition Fund, the Health Policy Research Program and the National Forum on Health, the Primary Health Care Transition Fund, and the Canadian Institutes of Health Research. It also provides information about the wide range of projects undertaken or sponsored by Health Canada.

http://www.hc-sc.gc.ca/english/protection/research.html

The Deutsche Gesellschaft Ttechnische Zusammenarbeit is a government-owned corporation for international cooperation that provides information about innovative approaches to reproductive health through peer education, a youth center, theater, action research, and community-based services.

http://www.gtz.de/srh/english/project/proj3–4.html

Community Health

The Institute of Action Research for Community Health at the Indiana University School of Nursing, where the World Health Organization Collaborating Center in Healthy Cities is also located, seeks to promote, develop, and conduct interdisciplinary research relevant to community health. Services include consultation and technical assistance, action research, evaluation research, and healthy cities resources. The site provides a list of informative websites pertaining to Healthy Cities and Communities.

http://www.iupui.edu/~citynet/6.htm

The Community Health Research Unit site links people to the wide range of resources available through the Department of Epidemiology and Community Medicine at the University of Ottowa.

http://www.uottawa.ca/academic/med/epid/chru_eng.htm

International Organizations

The World Health Organization home page.

http://www.who.int/home-page/

The World Resources Institute is concerned largely with environmental issues related to population health and human well-being. It provides information, ideas, and solutions to global environmental problems.

http://www.wri.org/health/

SHARED (Scientists for Health and Research for Development) uses internet networks to share essential information on health research and development for developing countries. It provides access to people, projects, organizations, electronic journals, other databases, networks, and groups.

http://www.shared.de/default.asp

Health Education Library for People (HELP), a non-profit organization, provides health education resources for people in India. Includes on-line resources for action research in holistic health (http://www.healthlibrary.com/reading/banyanIII/ chap2.htm).

http://www.healthlibrary.com

Alcohol and Drugs

U.S. National Clearinghouse for Alcohol and Drug Information provides informative research briefs focusing on the use of community action research related to the prevention of alcohol and other drug problems.

http://www.health.org/research/res-brf/

Mental Health

ARA Mental Health Action Research and Advocacy Association of Greater Vancouver, Canada, promotes direct advocacy services that encourage the balanced well-being of individuals in order to achieve a normal, productive life. The research division presents project reports focusing on a wide range of issues, including income assistance, housing, medications, employment, and crisis intervention. The site provides links to other mental health sites for Canada and the United States.

http://home.istar.ca/~mha_adv/

The U.S. National Institute of Mental Health home site provides a wide range of resources for the public, practitioners, and researchers. It includes mental disorder information, as well as research fact sheets, conference reports, research reports, funding opportunities, and patient education materials.

http://www.nimh.nih.gov/

Health Promotion

The Alberta Consortium for Health Promotion Research and Education site provides on-line access to health promotion and injury prevention information in Alberta, Canada.

http://www.health-in-action.org/new/Consort/consort.shtml

HIV

The Health Action Research Team provides programs and resources to enhance the quality of life for HIV-infected and affected youth through peer-based skill building, education, training, and support.

http://www.themeasurementgroup.com/resource/hart_broch.htm

University Programs

Action Research

A site maintained by the University of California San Francisco sponsors communities of teachers and scientists to examine teaching and learning to improve classroom practice with respect to issues such as equity, language, acquisition, and conceptual development in science.

http:/ /www.ucsf.edu/sep/action.html

The following incorporate links to health and science mentorship programs.

http:/ /www.ucsf.edu/sep/mentor.html

http:/ /www.ucsf.edu/sep/bioteach.html

Participatory Action Research in Public Health includes a course outline from the University of California San Francisco that provides an interesting list of reading resources.

http:/ /www.futurehealth.ucsf.edu/pdf_files/_PH_219C_2002revised.pdf

The University of Sydney Faculty of Health Sciences, containing information about courses for Improving Health Systems courses, includes a virtual library comprising sites for action research, e-reports, an action research electronic reader, and web links.

Research and cooperation activities focus on improving health systems, cyberspace, cooperation, and international health with an associated e-mail discussion list.

http:/ /casino.cchs.usyd.edu.au/arow/

The Center for Action Research in Professional Practice at the University of Bath School of Management provides a wide range of information on action research, including papers and publications, conferences and workshops, and related websites.

http:/ /www.bath.ac.uk/carpp/carpp.htm

References

Abbott, P., & Sapsford, R. (Eds.). (1997). *Research into practice: A reader for nurses and the caring professions*. Buckingham, UK: Open University Press.

Aboriginal Legal Service. (1994). *Counting the cost: Policing in Wiluna 1994*. Aboriginal Legal Service of Western Australia, Perth.

Allamani, A., Forni, E., Ammannati, P., Sani, I., & Centurioni, A. (2000). Alcohol carousel and children's school drawings as part of a community education strategy. In *Substance Use & Misuse*. Florence Health Agency, Integrated Alcohol Center, Florence, Italy. 35(1&2):125–139

Allen, D. (2000). *The changing shape of nursing practice: The role of nurses in the hospital division of labour*. London: Routledge.

Altheide, D., & Johnson, J. (1998). Criteria for assessing interpretive validity in qualitative research. In N. K. Denzin & Y. S. Lincoln (Eds.), *Collecting and interpreting qualitative materials*. Thousand Oaks, CA: Sage.

Arhar, J., Holly, M. L., & Kastern, H. (2000). *Action research for teachers: Traveling the yellow brick road*. Upper Saddle River, NJ: Pearson Education.

Arnett, R. (1986). *Communication and community*. Carbondale, IL: Southern Illinois University Press.

Atkinson, P. (1992). *Understanding ethnographic texts*. Newbury Park, CA: Sage.

Barbour, S, & Kitzinger, J. (Eds.). (1998). *Developing focus group research: Politics, theory and practice*. Thousand Oaks, CA: Sage.

Barker, S., & Barker, R. (1994). Managing change in an interdisciplinary inpatient unit: An action research approach. *Journal of Mental Health Administration*, Winter.

Barrett, P. (2001). The early mothering project: What happened when the words "action research" came to life for a group of midwives. In P. Reason & H. Bradbury (Eds.), *Handbook of action research*. Thousand Oaks, CA: Sage.

Barthes, R. (1986). *The rustle of language* (R. Howard, Trans.). New York: Hill and Wang

Baudrillard, J. (1983). *Simulations*. New York: Foreign Agent Press.

Bell, J. (1993). *Doing your research project: A guide for first-time researchers in education and social science*. Buckingham: Open University Press.

Benner, P. (1994). *Interpretive phenomenology: Embodiment, caring, and ethics in health and illness*. Thousand Oaks, CA: Sage.

Benner, P., Janson-Bjerklie, S., Ferketich, S., & Becker, G. (1994). Moral dimensions of living with a chronic illness: Autonomy, responsibility, and the limits of control. In P. Benner (Ed.), *Interpretive phenomenology*. Thousand Oaks, CA: Sage.

Berge, B-M., & Ve, H. (2000). *Action research for gender equity*. Buckingham, UK: Open University Press.

Berger, P., & Luckmann, T. (1967). *The social construction of reality: A treatise in the sociology of knowledge*. New York: Anchor.

Berger, P., Berger, B., & Kellner, H. (1973). *The homeless mind: Modernization and consciousness*. New York: Random House.

Block, P. (1990). *The empowered manager: Positive political skills at work*. San Francisco: Jossey Bass.

Boeckh, P. (1968). *On interpretation and criticism* (J. Pritchard, Trans. and Ed.). Norman, OK: University of Oklahoma Press.

Bogdan, R., & Biklen, S. (1992). *Qualitative research for education*. Boston: Allyn and Bacon.

Bond, M. (1999). Placing poverty on the agenda of the primary health care team: An evaluation of an action research project. *Health and Social Care in the Community, 7*(1), 9–16.

Bray, J., Lee, L., Smith, S., & Yorks, L. (Eds.). (2000). *Collaborative inquiry in practice: Action, reflection, and making meaning*. Thousand Oaks, CA: Sage.

Brown, A., & Dowling, P. (1998). *Doing research/reading research. A mode of interrogation for education*. London: Falmer.

Brown, M., Koch T., & Webb, C. (2000). Information needs of women with non-invasive breast cancer. *Journal of Clinical Nursing, 9*, 713–722.

Brown, R. (1992). Max van Manen and pedagogical human science research. In W. Pinar & W. Reynolds (Eds.), *Understanding curriculum as phenomenological and deconstructed text*. New York: Teachers College Press.

Bruner, E. (1986). Experience and its expressions. In V. Turner & E. Bruner (Eds.), *The anthropology of experience*. Urbana, IL: University of Illinois Press.

Buber, M. (1958). *I and thou*. New York: Charles Scribner's Sons

Buber, M. (1969). *A believing humanism*. New York: Simon and Schuster.

Butler, P., & Cass, S. (Eds.). (1993). *Case studies of community development in health*. Northcote, Vic.: Centre for Development and Innovation in Health.

Bytheway, B., Bacigalupo, V., Bomat, J., Johnson, J., & Spart, S. (2001). *Understanding care, welfare and community: A reader*. New York: Routledge.

Calhoun, E. (1993). Action research: Three approaches. *Educational Leadership,* October.

Carr, W., & Kemmis, S. (1986). *Becoming critical: Education, knowledge, and action research*. Philadelphia: Falmer Press.

Carson, T., & Sumara, D. (Eds.). (1997). *Action research as a living practice*. New York: Peter Lang.

Chambers, R. (1992). Rapid but relaxed and participatory rural appraisal: Towards applications in health and nutrition. In N. Scrimshaw & G. Gleason (Eds.), *RAP Rapid assessment procedures. Qualitative methodologies for planning and evaluation of health related programs*. Boston: International Nutrition Foundation for Developing Countries.

Chesla, C. (1994). Parents caring practices with schizophrenic offspring. In P. Benner (Ed.), *Interpretive phenomenology*. Thousand Oaks, CA: Sage.

Chirban, J. (1996). *Interviewing in depth: The interactive-relational approach*. Thousand Oaks, CA: Sage

Christiansen, H., Goulet, L., Krentz, C., & Maeers, M. (Eds.). (1997). *Recreating relationships: Collaboration and educational reform*. Albany, NY: SUNY Press.

Clifford, J. (1988). *The predicament of culture*. Cambridge, MA: Harvard University Press.

Clifford, J., & Marcus, G. (Eds.). (1986). *Writing culture: The poetics and politics of ethnography*. Berkeley: University of California Press.

Cohen, E., & Casta, T. (1993). *Nursing case management*. St. Louis, MO: Mosby.

Community Development in Health Project. (1988). *Community development in health: A resources collection*. Northcote, Vic: District Health Council.

Cook, T., & Campbell, D. (1979). *Quasi-experimentation: Design and analysis for field settings*. Chicago: Rand McNally.

Coughlan, D., & Brannick, T. (2001). *Doing action research in your own organization*. Thousand Oaks, CA: Sage.

Couto, R., & Guthrie, C. (1999). *Making democracy work better: Mediating structure, social capital, and the democratic prospect*. Chapel Hill, NC: University of North Carolina Press.

Creswell, J. (2002). *Educational research: Planning, conducting and evaluating quantitative and qualitative research*. Upper Saddle River, NJ: Pearson.

Darbyshire, P. (1994). Parenting in public: Parental participation and involvement in the care of their hospitalized children. In P. Benner (Ed.), *Interpretive phenomenology*. Thousand Oaks, CA: Sage.

Darling-Hammond, L., & McLauglin, M. (1995). Policies that support professional development in an era of reform. *Phi Delta Kappan, 76*(8), 597–604.

Davies, P., & Gribben, J. (1991). *The matter myth: Beyond chaos and complexity*. London: Penguin.

Dedobbeleer, N., & Desjardins, S. (2001). Outcomes of an ecological and participatory approach to prevent alcohol and other drug "abuse" among multiethnic adolescents. In *Substance Use & Misuse, 36*(13), 1959–1991.

deLaine, M. (2000). *Fieldwork, participation and practice: Ethics and dilemmas in qualitative research*. Thousand Oaks, CA: Sage.

deMarrais, K. B. (Ed.). (1998). *Inside stories: Qualitative research reflections*. Mahwah, NJ: Lawrence Erlbaum Associates.

Denzin, N. K. (1989a). *Interpretive biography*. Thousand Oaks, CA: Sage

Denzin, N. K. (1989b). *Interpretive interactionism*. Newbury Park, CA: Sage.

Denzin, N. K. (1997). *Interpretive ethnography*. Thousand Oaks, CA: Sage.

Denzin, N. K., & Lincoln, Y. S. (Eds.). (1994). *Handbook of qualitative research*. Thousand Oaks, CA: Sage.

Denzin, N. K., & Lincoln, Y. S. (Eds.). (1998a). *Collecting and interpreting qualitative materials*. Thousand Oaks, CA: Sage.

Denzin, N. K., & Lincoln, Y. S. (Eds.). (1998b). *The landscape of qualitative research: Theories and issues*. Thousand Oaks, CA: Sage.

Denzin, N. K., & Lincoln, Y. S. (Eds.). (2000). *Handbook of qualitative research* (2nd ed.). Thousand Oaks, CA: Sage.

Derrida, J. (1976). *Of grammatology*. Baltimore, MD: Johns Hopkins University Press.

Derrida, J. (1978). *Writing and difference*. Chicago: University of Chicago Press.

Deshler, D. (1990). Conceptual mapping: Drawing charts of the mind. In J. Mezirow & Associates (Eds.), *Fostering critical reflection in adulthood* (pp. 336–353). San Francisco: Jossey-Bass.

Dewey, J. (1916/1966). *Democracy in education*. New York: Macmillan.

Dilthey, W. (1976). *Selected writings*. Cambridge, UK: Cambridge University Press.

Dodds, J. (1995). Collaborative group inquiry—a blend of research and therapy. *Australian Social Work, 48*(3).

Dodds, J. (1997). *Cancer as bad luck or warning symbol: Constructed meanings of illness and healing*. Unpublished doctoral dissertation, University of Western Australia.

Doolittle, N. (1994). A clinical ethnography of stroke recovery. In P. Benner (Ed.), *Interpretive phenomenology*. Thousand Oaks, CA: Sage.

East, L., & Robinson, A. (1994). Change in process: Bringing about change in health care through action research. *Journal of Clinical Nursing, 3*, 57–61.

Eastwood, S., Kralik, D., & Koch, T. (2002). Compromising and containing: Self-management strategies used by men and women who live with multiple sclerosis and urinary incontinence. *Australian Journal of Holistic Nursing, 9(1)*: 33–43.

Edwards, C., Gandini, L., & Forman, G. (1998). *The hundred languages of children: The Reggio Amelia Approach—Advanced Reflections*. Greenwich, CT: Ablex.

Fals-Borda, O., & Rahman, M. (1991). *Action and knowledge: Breaking the monopoly with participatory action research*. New York: Apex.

Feiman-Nemser, S. (2000). *From preparation to practice: Designing a continuum to strengthen and sustain teaching*. Unpublished manuscript, Michigan State University.

Fink, A. (1995). *The survey handbook*. Thousand Oaks, CA: Sage.

Foucault, M. (1972). *The archaeology of knowledge*. New York: Random House.

Foucault, M. (1979). *Discipline and punish: The birth of the prison*. New York: Random House.

Foucault, M. (1984). *The Foucault reader* (P. Rabinow, Ed.). Harmondworth, UK: Penguin.

Friedman, M. (1974). *The hidden human image*. New York: Dell Publishing.

Friedman, M. (1983). *The confirmation of otherness: in family, community, and society*. New York: Pilgrim Press.

Frus, P. (1994). *The politics and poetics of journalistic narrative*. New York: Cambridge University Press.

Fuller, R., & Petch, A. (1995). *Practitioner research*. Buckingham, UK: Open University Press.

Gadamer, H-G. (1980). *Dialogue and dialectic: Eight hermeneutical studies on Plato* (P. Smith, Trans.). New Haven: Yale University Press.

Garfinkel, H. (1967). *Studies in ethnomethodology*. Englewood Cliffs, NJ: Prentice Hall.

Genat, W. (2001). *Aboriginal health workers: Beyond the clinic, beyond the rhetoric*. Unpublished doctoral dissertation, University of Western Australia.

Glaser, B., & Strauss, A. (1976). *The discovery of grounded theory: Strategies for qualitative research*. Chicago, IL: Aldine.

Goffman, E. (1961). *Asylums: Essays on the social situation of mental patients and other inmates*. New York: Anchor.

Goodenough, W. (1971). *Culture, language and society*. Reading, MA: Addison-Wesley.

Gordon, D. (1994). The ethics of ambiguity and concealment around cancer: Interpretations through a local Italian world. In P. Benner (Ed.), *Interpretive phenomenology*. Thousand Oaks, CA: Sage.

Graham, K., & Chandler-Coutts, M. (2000). Community action research: Who does what to whom and why? Lessons learned from local prevention efforts (international experiences). In *Substance Use & Misuse, 35*(1&2): 87–110.

Graue, M., & Walsh, D. (1998). *Studying children in context: Theories, methods, and ethics*. Thousand Oaks, CA: Sage.

Green, L., George, M., Daniel, M., Frankish, C., Herbert, C., Bowie, W., & O'Neill, M. (1995). *Study of participatory research in health promotion*. Toronto: Royal Society of Canada.

Greenbaum T. (Ed.). (2000). *Moderating focus groups: A practical guide for group facilitation*. Thousand Oaks, CA: Sage.

Guba, E. G., & Lincoln, Y. S. (1989). *Fourth generation evaluation*. Newbury Park, CA: Sage.

Habermas, J. (1979). *Communication and the evolution of society* (T. McCarthy, Trans.). Boston: Beacon.

Haraway, D. (1988). "Situated knowledge: The Science question in feminism and the privilege of partial perspective." *Feminist Studies, 14*(3), 575–599.

Hart, E., & Bond, M. (1995). *Action research for health and social care: A guide to practice*. Buckingham, UK: Open University Press.

Harvey, D. (1989). *The condition of postmodernity: An enquiry into the origins of cultural change*. Cambridge, MA: Basil Blackwell

Hawley, W., & Valli, L. (1999). The essentials of effective professional development: A new consensus. In L. Darling-Hammond & G. Sykes (Eds.), *Teaching as the learning profession: A handbook of policy and practice*. San Francisco: Jossey-Bass.

Heath, S. (1983). *Ways with words: Language, life and work in communities and classrooms*. Cambridge, UK: Cambridge University Press.

Heidegger, M. (1962). *Being and time* (J. Macquarie and E. Robinson, Trans.). New York: Harper & Row.

Helm, J. (1999). Projects: Exploring children's interests. *Scholastic Early Childhood Today,* March.

Heron, J. (1996) *Co-operative inquiry: Research into the human condition*. London: Sage.

Hills, M. (2001). Using co-operative inquiry to transform evaluation of nursing students' clinical practice. In P. Reason & H. Bradbury (Ed.), *Handbook of action research*. Thousand Oaks, CA: Sage.

Holder, H., & Moore, R. (2000). *Substance Use & Misuse*. Prevention Research Center, Berkeley, California, USA. *35*(1&2):75–86.

Holstein, J., & Gubrium, J. (1995). *The active interview*. Thousand Oaks, CA: Sage.

Holter, I., & Schwartz-Barcott, D. (1993). Action research: What is it and how has it been used in nursing? *Journal of Advanced Nursing, 18*, 298–304.

Horowitz, I. (1970). Sociological snoopers and journalistic moralizers. *Transaction, 7*, 4–8.

Huffman, J. (1997). *Beyond TQM: Tools & techniques for high performance improvement*. Sunnyvale, CA: Lanchester Press.

Husserl, E. (1970). *Logical investigation*. New York: Humanities Press.

Husserl, E. (1976). *Logical investigations* (J. Findlay, Trans.). New York: The Humanities Press.

Huyssens, A. (1986). *After the great divide: Modernism, mass culture, postmodernism*. Bloomington, IA: Indiana University Press.

Iyer, P., Taptich, B., & Bernocchi-Losey, D. (1991). *Nursing process and nursing diagnosis*. Philadelphia, PA: W.B. Saunders.

Jackson, M. (1996). *Things as they are: New directions in phenomenological anthropology*. Bloomington, IN: Indiana University Press.

Johnson, B. (2001). Toward a new classification of non-experimental quantitative research. *Educational Researcher, 30*(2).

Johnson, G. (1995). *Fire in the mind: Science, faith and the search for order*. New York: Vintage Books.

Komaromy, C. (Ed.). (2001). *Dilemmas in U.K. health care*. Buckingham, UK: Open University Press.

Kelly, A., & Sewell, S. (1988). *With head, heart, and hand*. Brisbane, Australia: Boolarong.

Kemmis, S., & McTaggart, R. (1988). *The action research planner*. Geelong, Australia: Deakin University Press.

Kent, J. (2000). *Social perspectives on pregnancy and childbirth for midwives, nurses and the caring professions*. Open University Press.

Kickett, D., McCauley, D., & Stringer, E. (1986). *Community development processes: An introductory handbook*. Perth, Australia: Curtin University of Technology.

Kincheloe, J., & McClaren, P. (1994). Rethinking critical theory and qualitative research. In N. Denzin & Y. Lincoln (Eds.), *Handbook of qualitative research*. Thousand Oaks, CA: Sage.

Koch, T., & Kelly, S. (1999). Understanding what is important for women who live with multiple sclerosis. *The Australian Journal of Holistic Nursing, 8(1):* 4–13.

Koch, T., & Kralik, D. (2001a). Chronic illness: Reflections on a community-based action research program. *Journal of Advanced Nursing, 36* (1), 23–31.

Koch, T., & Kralik, D. (2001b). Reflections on a community-based action research program. *Journal of Advanced Nursing, 36*(1), 23–31.

Koch, T., Kralik, D., & Kelly, S. (2000). "We just don't talk about it": Men living with urinary incontinence and multiple sclerosis. *International Journal of Nursing Practice, 6*, 253–260.

Koch, T., Kralik, D., Eastwood, S., & Schofield, A. (2001). Breaking the silence: Women living with multiple sclerosis and urinary incontinence. *International Journal of Nursing Practice, 7*, 16–23.

Koch, T., Kralik, D., & Sonnack, D. (2000). Women living with type two diabetes: The intrusion of illness. *Journal of Clinical Nursing, 8*(6), 712–722.

Koch, T., Kralik, D., & Taylor, J. (2000). Men living with diabetes: Minimizing the intrusiveness of the disease. *Journal of Clinical Nursing, 9*, 247–254.

Koch, T., Selim, P. & Kralich, D. (2001). Enhancing lives through the development of a community based participatory action research program. *Journal of Clinical Nursing, 11:* 109–117.

Koch, T., Selim, P., & Kralik, D. (2002). Enhancing lives through the development of a community based participatory action research program. *Journal of Clinical Nursing, 11*, 109–117.

Kralik, D., Koch, T., & Telford, K. (2001). Constructions of sexuality for midlife women living with chronic illness. *Journal of Advanced Nursing, 35*(2): 180–187.

Komaromy, C. (2001). *Dilemmas in UK health care.* Buckingham, UK: Open University Press.

Kretzmann, J., & McKnight, J. (1993). *Building communities from the inside out: A path toward finding and mobilizing a community's assets.* Chicago: ACTA Publications.

Krueger, R. (1994). *Focus groups: A practical guide for applied research* (2nd ed.). Thousand Oaks, CA: Sage.

Krueger, R. (1997a). *Moderating focus groups.* Thousand Oaks, CA: Sage.

Krueger, R. (1997b). *Developing questions for focus groups.* Thousand Oaks, CA: Sage.

Krueger, R., & Casey, M. (2000). *Focus groups: A practical guide for applied research* (3rd ed.). Newbury Park: Sage.

Kvale, S. (1996). *Interviews: An introduction to qualitative research interviewing.* Thousand Oaks, CA: Sage.

Lather, P. (1993). Fertile obsession: Validity after post-structuralism. *Sociological Quarterly, 35.*

Lewin, G., & Lewin, K. (1942). Democracy and the school. *Understanding the Child, 10*, 7–11.

Lewin, K. (1938). Experiments on autocratic and democratic principles. *Social Frontier, 4*, 316–319.

Lewin, K. (1946). Action research and minority problems. *Journal of Social Issues, 2*(4), 34–46.

Lewin, K. (1948). *Resolving social conflicts.* New York: Harper.

Lincoln, Y., & Guba, E. (1985). *Naturalistic inquiry.* Newbury Park, CA: Sage.

Lupton, C., Peckham, S., & Taylor, P. (1998). *Managing public involvement in health care purchasing.* Buckingham, UK: Open University Press.

Lyotard, J-F. (1984). *The postmodern condition: A report on knowledge.* Minneapolis: University of Minnesota Press.

Makay, J. (1972). *The rhetorical dialogue.* Dubuque, IA: William C. Brown.

Malinowski, B. (1922/1961). *Argonauts of the Western Pacific.* New York: E.P. Dutton.

Maltrud, K., Polacsek, M., & Wallerstein, N. (1997). *Participatory evaluation workbook for community initiatives.* Albuquerque, NM: University of New Mexico School of Medicine.

Marcus, G. (1986). *Anthropology as cultural critique: An experimental moment in the human sciences.* Chicago: University of Chicago Press.

Marcus, G. (1998). *Ethnography through thick and thin.* Princeton, NJ: Princeton University Press.

Marshall, C., & Rossman, G. (1999). *Designing qualitative research* (3rd ed.). Thousand Oaks, CA: Sage.

Mascarenhas, J. (1992). Participatory rural appraisal and participatory learning methods: Recent experiences from MYRADA and South India. In N. Scrimshaw & G. Gleason (Eds.). *RAP Rapid assessment procedures qualitative methodologies for planning and evaluation of health related programs.* Boston: International Nutrition Foundation for Developing Countries.

Mash, B., & Meulenberg-Buskens, I. (2001). 'Holding it lightly'—The co-operative inquiry group: A method for developing educational materials. *Medical Education, 35*, 1108–1114.

McCracken, G. (1988). *The long interview.* Thousand Oaks, CA: Sage. Grant

McElroy, A., & Shepherd, G. (1999). The assessment and management of self-harming patients in an accident and emergency department. *Journal of Clinical Nursing, 8,* 66–72.

McEwan, P. (2000). The potential impact of large-scale voucher programs. *Review of Educational Research, 70*(2).

McLean, J. (1995). *Improving education through action research: A guide for administrators and teachers.* Thousand Oaks, CA: Corwin.

McNiff, J. (1995). *Action research principles and practice.* New York: Routledge.

McNiff, J., Lomax, P., & Whitehead, J. (1996). *You and your action research project.* Bournemouth, UK: Hyde.

McTaggart, R. (Ed.). (1997). *Participatory action research: International contexts and consequences.* Albany, NY: SUNY Press.

McWhinney, I. (1989). *A textbook of family medicine.* New York: Oxford University Press.

Mead, G. (1934). *Mind, self and society.* Chicago: University of Chicago Press.

Meerdink, J. (1999). Driving a car for the first time: Teachers, caregivers and a child-driven approach. *Early Childhood Matters: The Bulletin of the Bernard Van Leer Foundation, 91.*

Menon, M. (1993). A tea trolley support service in a hospital oncology clinic. In P. Butler & S. Cass (Eds.), *Case studies of community development in health.* Melbourne: Centre for the Development of Innovation in Health.

Merchant, B., & Ingram Willis, A. (Eds.). (2001). *Multiple and intersecting identities in qualitative research.* Mahwah, NJ: Lawrence Erlbaum Associates.

Meriam-Webster Online Dictionary. (2001). www.m-w.com

Mienczakowski, J., & Morgan, S. (2001). Ethnodrama: Constructing participatory, experiential, and compelling action research through performance. In P. Reason & H. Bradbury (Eds.), *Handbook of action research.* Thousand Oaks, CA: Sage.

Milgram, S. (1963). Behavioral study of obedience. *Journal of Abnormal and Social Psychology, 67,* 371–378.

Mills, C. W. (1959). *The sociological imagination.* New York: Oxford.

Mills, G. (2000). *Action research: A guide for the teacher researcher.* Columbus, OH: Merrill/Prentice Hall.

Moon, G., Gould, M., & Colleagues (2000). *Epidemiology: An introduction.* Buckingham, UK: Open University Press.

Morgan, D. (1997a). *Planning focus groups.* Thousand Oaks, CA: Sage

Morgan, D. (1997b). *The focus group guidebook.* Thousand Oaks, CA: Sage.

Morgan, D., & Krueger, R. (1997). *The focus group kit: Volumes 1–6.* Thousand Oaks, CA: Sage.

Moyer, A., Coristine, M., Jamault, M., Roberge, G., & O'Hagan, M. (1999). Identifying older people in need using action research. *Journal of Clinical Nursing, 8,* 103–111.

Mueller-Vollmer, K. (Ed.). (1985). *The hermeneutics reader.* New York: Continuum.

Nietszche, F. (1979). *On truth and lies in a nonmoral sense. Philosophy and truth: Selections from Nietzsche's notebooks in the early 1870s.* Atlantic City, NJ: Humanities Press.

Noffke, S. (1997). Professional, personal and political dimensions of action research. *Review of Educational Research, 22.* Washington, DC: AERA.

Oleson, V. (1993). Unfinished business: The problematics of women, health and healing. *The Science of Caring, 5,* 3–6.

Oleson, V. (1998). Feminisms and models of qualitative research. In N. Denzin & Y. Lincoln (Eds.), *The landscape of qualitative research.* Thousand Oaks, CA: Sage.

Oliver, S., & Peersman, G. (2001). *Using research for effective health promotion.* Buckingham, UK: Open University Press.

Oppenheim, A. (1966). *Questionnaire design and attitude measurement.* London: Heinemann.

Patton, M. (1990). *Qualitative evaluation and research methods* (2nd ed.). Newbury Park, CA: Sage.

Persig, R. (1974). *Zen and the art of motorcycle maintenance.* New York: Bantam.

Petty, R. (1997). Everything is different now: Surviving ethnographic research. In E. Stringer et al. (Eds.), *Community based ethnography: Breaking traditional boundaries of research, teaching and learning.* Mahwah, NJ: Lawrence Erlbaum.

Pratiss, J. (Ed.). (1985). *Reflections: The anthropological muse.* Washington, DC: American Anthropological Association.

Punch, M. (1994). Politics and ethics in qualitative research. In N. Denzin & Y. Lincoln (Eds.), *Handbook of qualitative research.* Thousand Oaks, CA: Sage.

Rabinow, P., & Sullivan, W. (Eds.). (1987). *Interpretive social science: A second look* (2nd ed.). Berkeley: University of California Press.

Reason, P., & Bradbury, H. (2001). *Handbook of action research*. Thousand Oaks, CA: Sage.

Reason, P., & Bradbury, H. (2002). Action research: Purpose, vision, mission. Unpublished dialogue.

Ricoeur, P. (1979). The model of the text: Meaningful action considered as a text. In P. Rabinow & W. Sullivan (Eds.), *Interpretive social science*. Berkeley: University of California Press.

Rogers, A., Hassell, K., & Nicolaas, G., (1998). *Demanding patients?* Buckingham, UK: Open University Press.

Rorty, R. (1989). *Contigiency, irony, and solidarity*. Cambridge, UK: Cambridge University Press.

Rose, K., Waterman, H., Mcleod, D., & Tullo, A. (1999). Planning and managing research into day surgery for cataract. *Journal of Advanced Nursing, 29*(6), 1514–1519.

Rosenau, P. (1992). *Postmodernism and the social sciences: Insights, inroads and intrusions*. Princeton, NJ: Princeton University Press.

Ross, F., & MacKenzie, A. (1996). *Nursing in primary health care: Policy into practice*. London: Routledge.

Rubin, H., & Rubin, I. (1995). *Qualitative interviewing: The art of hearing data*. Thousand Oaks, CA: Sage.

Scheurich, J. (1992). The paradigmatic transgressions of validity. Unpublished manuscript. Quoted in Denzin, N. and Y. Lincoln (Eds.), *Handbook of qualitative research*. Thousand Oaks, CA: Sage.

Schmuck, R. (1997). *Practical action research for change*. Arlington Heights, IL: IRI/Skylight Training and Publishing.

Schouten, D., & Watling, R. (1997). *Media action projects: A model for integrating video in project-based education, training and community development*. Nottingham, UK: University of Nottingham Urban Programme Research Group.

Schutz, A. (1964). *Studies in social theory*. The Hague: Martinus Nijhoff.

Schutz, A. (1970). *On phenomenology and social relations*. Chicago, IL: Chicago University Press.

Seale, C., Pattison, S., & Davey, B. (2001). *Medical knowledge: Doubt and certainty*. Buckingham, UK: Open University Press.

Selekman, M. (1997). *Solution-focused therapy with children*. New York: Guilford Press.

Selim, P., Bashford, C., & Grossman, C. (2001). Evidence-based practice: Tap water cleansing of leg ulcers in the community. *Journal of Clinical Nursing, 10*, 372–379.

Senge, P., Kleiner, A., Roberts, C., Ross, R., & Smith, B. (1994). *The fifth discipline fieldbook*. Doubleday.

Sieber, J. (1992). *Planning ethically responsible research*. Newbury Park, CA: Sage.

Silverman, D. (2000). *Doing qualitative research. A practical handbook*. Thousand Oaks, CA: Sage.

Smithbattle, L. (1994). Beyond normalizing: The role of narrative in understanding teenage mothers' transition to mothering. In P. Benner (Ed.), *Interpretive phenomenology*. Thousand Oaks, CA: Sage.

Spencer, S., Unsworth, J., & Burke, W. (Eds.). (2001). *Developing community nursing practice*. Buckingham, UK: Open University Press.

Spradley, J. (1979a). *The ethnographic interview*. New York: Holt, Rinehart and Winston.

Spradley, J. (1979b). *Participant observation*. New York: Holt, Rinehart and Winston.

Spradley, J., & McCurdy, D. (1972). *The cultural experience*. Prospect Heights, IL: Waveland Press.

Stake, R. (1994). Case studies. In N. Denzin & Y. Lincoln (Eds.), *The handbook of qualitative research*. Thousand Oaks, CA: Sage.

Stein, M., Smith, M., & Silver, E. (1999). The development of professional developers: Learning to assist teachers in new settings in new ways. *Harvard Education Review, 69*(3).

St Leger, A., & Walsworth-Bell, J. (1999). *Change-promoting research for health services: A guide for resource managers, research and development commissioners and researchers*. Buckingham, UK: Open University Press.

Strauss, A., & Corbin, J. (1994). Grounded theory: An overview. In N. Denzin and Y. Lincoln (Eds.), *Handbook of qualitative research*. Thousand Oaks, CA: Sage.

Street, A. (Ed.). (1995). *Establishing a participatory action research group in nursing replay: Researching nursing culture together* (Vol. 1, 1st ed.). Melbourne: Churchill Livingston.

Stringer, E. (1996). *Action research: A handbook for practitioners*. Thousand Oaks, CA: Sage.

Stringer, E. (1997). *Community based ethnography: Breaking traditional boundaries of research, teaching and learning*. Mahwah, NJ: Lawrence Erlbaum.

Stringer, E. (1999). *Action research* (2nd ed.). Thousand Oaks, CA: Sage.

Stringer, E., & Genat, W. (1998). *The double helix of action research*. Qualitative Research in Education Conference, Athens, Georgia.

Stuhlmiller, C. (1994). Narrative methodology in disaster studies: Rescuers of Cypress. In P. Benner (Ed.), *Interpretive phenomenology: Embodiment, caring and ethics in health and illness.* Thousand Oaks, CA: Sage.

Tarnas, R. (1991). *The passion of the western mind.* London: Crown.

Taylor, B. (2000). *Reflective practice: A guide for nurses and midwives.* Buckingham, UK: Open University Press.

Tennant, G. (2001). *Six sigma: SPC and TQM in manufacturing and services.* Aldershol, UK: Gower Publishing.

Toombs, S. (1993). *The meaning of illness: A phenomenological account of the different perspectives of physician and patient.* Boston: Kluwer Academic Publishers.

Trinh, T. (1991). *When the moon waxes red: Representation, gender and cultural politics.* New York: Routledge.

Tyler, S. (1986). Post-modern ethnography: From document of the occult to occult document. In J.Clifford & G. Marcus (Eds.), *Writing culture.* Berkeley, CA: University of California Press.

UNICEF. (1978). Report of the International Conference on Primary Health Care, Alma-Ata, USSR, September 6–12. Geneva, ICPHC/ALA/78.10.

Van Manen, M. (1977). The phenomenology of pedagogic observation. *Canadian Journal of Education, 4*(1), 5–16.

Van Manen, M. (1982). Phenomenological pedagogy. *Curriculum Inquiry, 12*(3), 283–299.

Van Manen, M. (1984). Practising phenomenological writing. *Phenomenology and Pedagogy, 2*(1), 36–39.

Van Manen, M. (1988). The relation between research and pedagogy. In W. F. Pinar (Ed.), *Contemporary curriculum discourses* (pp. 437–452). Scottsdale, AZ: Gorsuch Scarisbrick.

Van Manen, M. (1990). *Researching lived experience: Human science for an action sensitive pedagogy.* London, Ontario: Althouse Press

Van Willigan, J. (1993). *Applied anthropology: An introduction.* Westport, CN: Bergin and Garvey.

Wadsworth, Y. (2001). The mirror, the magnifying glass, the compass and the map: Facilitating participatory action research. In P. Reason & H. Bradbury (Eds.), *Handbook of action research.* Thousand Oaks, CA: Sage.

Wadsworth, Y. (1997). *Everyday evaluation on the run* (2nd ed.). St Leonards, Australia: Allen & Unwin.

Wass, A. (2000). *Promoting health: The primary health care approach* (2nd ed.). New York: Harcourt.

Webb, C., & Koch, T. (1997). Women's experience of non-invasive breast cancer: Literature review and study report. *Journal of Advanced Nursing, 25,* 514–525.

Weis, L., & Fine, M. (2000). *Speed bumps: A student-friendly guide to qualitative research.* New York: Teachers College Press.

West, C. (1989). *The American evasion of philosophy.* Madison, WI: University of Wisconsin Press.

Whyte, D. (1997). *Explorations in family nursing.* London: Routledge.

Wicks, D. (1998). *Nurses and doctors at work: Rethinking professional boundaries.* Buckingham, UK: Open University Press.

Williams, A. (2000). *Nursing, medicine and primary care.* Buckingham, UK: Open University Press

Winter, R., & Munn-Giddings, C. (2001). *A handbook for action research in health and social care.* London: Routledge.

Wolcott, H. (1994). *Transforming qualitative data: Description, analysis and interpretation.* Thousand Oaks, CA: Sage.

Wong, K. (1993). The house party. In P. Butler & S. Cass (Eds.), *Case studies of community development in health.* Melbourne: Centre for the Development of Innovation in Health.

World Health Organization. (1978). Report of the international conference on primary health care, Alma-Ata, USSR, September 6–12, Geneva.

World Health Organization. (1986). Ottawa charter for health promotion–Report of the first international conference on health promotion, Ottawa. Geneva.

World Health Organization. (1988). The declaration of Alma Ata. *World Health,* August/September.

Wros, P. (1994). The ethical context of nursing care of dying patients in critical care. In P. Benner (Ed.), *Interpretive phenomenology.* Thousand Oaks, CA: Sage.

Young, S. (1999). *Negotiating racial boundaries and organizational borders: An interpretive study of a cross-cultural training programme.* Unpublished doctoral dissertation, University of Western Australia.

Youngman, M. (1982). Designing and analyzing questionnaires. In J. Bell (Ed.), *Conducting small-scale investigations in educational management.* London: Harper and Row.

Index

Entries in **bold** indicate a figure entry.

Abbott, P., 7
Accounts; *See* Written reports and
    accounts
Action agenda, and problem solving, 145
Action plan
  agenda, 145
  construction of, 145–146
  investigating alcohol issues, 168–169
  planning chart, **146**
  and problem solving, 144–147
  reviewing of, 146–147
  strategic planning, 159–160
  supervision of, 147
Action research; *See also* Research
  and alcohol use, 2
  alternative healing strategies, 2
  applications for, 2, 13–15
  approaches to, 16–26
  benchmarks and protocols, 2
  case studies, 162–182
  and changing health context, 12–13
  characteristics of, 5, 6–8
  and clinic, agency, or community
    relationships, 26–29
  communication in, 116–117
  and community care, 13
  conceptualized, 3
  conceptualized research, 3
  defined, 3
  engaging in heart, 34–35
  enlarging the circle of inquiry, 11
  human dimensions of, 32–35, **34**
  incontinence management processes,
    2, 8–9
  interpretive, 27–29, 30
  naturalistic inquiry, 20–26
  need for, 1
  and nursing practice changes, 13
  objective science approach, 16–20
  on-line resources, 183–189
  Participatory Action Research (PAR),
    8, 26, 29
  participatory processes of inquiry,
    9–10
  planning an design, 35–44
  processes of investigation, 28

and public involvement, 13
purpose of, 3
quality of, 48–49
reading of reports, 25–26
relationships, 26–29
renal disease, 2
research cycle, 4–5, **5**
research helix, 4–5, **5**
research spiral, 11
roles of participants, 10
sequence, 5, **6**
systematic inquiry, 28
systematic processes of inquiry,
    4–5, 28
transformational understanding, 3
trustworthiness, 49–53
validity of, 48–55
and western scientific knowledge, 13
work effectiveness, 1–2
working developmentally, 11–12
working principles, 55–56
Action Research Health Care
    Network, 186
Alcohol and Drugs, and Internet, 188
Alcohol, primary health care issues, 168
Allamani, A., 136
Allen, D., 13
Alma Ata Declaration on Primary
    Health Care (PHC), 28, 151
ALS, 168
Altheide, D., 53
Ammannati, P., 136
Arhar, J., 107
Artistic and dramatic performances,
    132–136
  alcohol education, 136
  community health needs survey, 135
  developing a script, 133
  domestic violence, 135
  examples of, 135–136
  frail-aged accommodation project, 136
  HIV awareness, 135
  planning a performance, 133
  producing of, 134
  video and electronic media,
    134–137

Atkinson, P., 132
Audio-visuals, and presentations,
    129–131
Audit review evaluation; *See* Evaluation
Australian Aboriginal people, 23–24
Autobiographies, 119–120

Bacigalupo, V., 13
Barbour, S., 70
Barker, R., 172, 173
Barker, S., 172, 173
Barrett, Penelope, 13, 144
Barthes, R., 21
Bashford, C., 178
Becker, G., 14
Benner, P., 14, 24
Berge, B-M., 7
Berger, Peter, 20
Bernocchi-Losey, 141
Biklen, S., 7, 107
Biographies, 119–120
Block, P., 157
Bogdan, R., 7, 107
Bomat, J., 13
Bond, M., 13, 174
Bradbury, H., 7
Brannick, T., 7, 157
Bray, J., 7
Bruner, E., 21
Bumpass Cove Citizens Group
    (BCCG), 166
Burke, W., 1, 7, 13
Butler, P., 152
Bytheway, B., 13

Cancer, and psychotherapy case study,
    164–165
Care, and research ethics, 45
Carr, S., 7
Carson, T., 7
Case study
  Action Research and Evidence-Based
    Wound Management, 178
  Acute Care Protocols in Accident and
    Emergency, 175
  change management, 172–173

creative prevention strategies, 167
Developing Clinical Protocols for
     Cataract Surgery, 177
Entry to Cross-Cultural Inquiry: The
     House Party, 181–182
Health Promotion and Community
     Development, 166
Incorporating the Social Context:
     Collaborative Reflection within a
     Family Practice, 174
Integrating the Isolated Aged into
     Community Practice, 176
managing incontinence, 8–9, 163
Oncology Clinic Tea Trolley, 180
Parent Participation with
     Hospitalized Child, 170–171
Primary Health Care: Investigating
     Alcohol Issues, 168–169
Psychotherapy: Focusing Client Self-
     Help Groups, 164–165
Self-Care Strategies in Community
     Nursing, 163
WHO Protocol: Stories of Family
     Physicians, 179
Casey, M., 70
Cass, S., 152
Casta, T., 141
Cataract surgery, protocols for, 177
Categorizing and coding, 103–108, **104**
  category system, 105–106
  frameworks for reports and
       accounts, 111
  organizing of, 107–108
  purposes and processes of, 103
  reviewing data sets, 104
  reviewing the research question,
       103–104
  subcategories, 108
  taxonomy, 105, **106**, 106–107
  unitizing the data, 105
Category system; *See* Categorizing and
     coding
Central tendencies, and Statistical and
     numerical data, 83
Centurioni, A., 136
Chambers, R., 73
Change management, 172–173
Chesla, C., 14
Chirban, J., 61, 66
Client care
  assessment, 141
  case management, 143
  diagnosis, 141
  evaluation, 142–143
  implementation, 142
  planning, 142

process of, 141–143
Client care, analysis, 141
Client case notes, and data gathering,
     79–80
Cohen, E., 141
Collective accounts, 121
Communication, 56
  academic, 118
  and action research, 116–117
  audiences for, 118
  forms of, 117–118
  organizational, 118
  professional, 118
  public, 118
Communication; *See also* Reports;
     Presentations; Written reports
     and accounts
Community care, 13
Community, creative prevention
     strategies, 167
Community development, 151–154
  consensus building strategies,
       152–153
  empowerment strategies, 153–154
  hazardous waste problems case
       study, 166
Community Development in Health
     Project, 152
Community health, and Internet, 187
Community nursing, self-care
     strategies, 163
Community organizations, and
     Internet, 186
Comparisons, and Statistical and
     numerical data, 83
Componential analysis, 105–107
Concept culture, 21
Confidentiality, and research ethics, 45
Consensus building strategies, 152–153
Continuous Quality Improvement
     (CQI), 141
Coristine, M., 176
Correlations, and Statistical and
     numerical data, 84
Coughlan, D., 7
Couto, R., 166
CQI; *See* Continuous Quality
     Improvement (CQI)
Credibility, 50–52
  diverse case analysis, 51
  member checks, 52
  participant debriefing, 51
  and persistent observation, 50–51
  prolonged engagement, 50
  referential adequacy, 51–52
  triangulation, 51

Creswell, J., 40, 41, 81, 95, 107
Culture; *See also* Human interaction

Darbyshire, P., 14, 170, 171
Data analysis, 44
  analyzing collaboratively, 111–113
  analyzing epiphanies, 91–102, **94**
  categorizing and coding, 103–108
  constructing conceptual frameworks,
       101–102
  developing collaborative accounts, 112
  enhancing analysis, 109–110
  epiphanies deconstruction, 98–100,
       99, 101–102
  epiphanies in observations and
       representations, 100
  expression of words, 96–97
  focus group analysis, **112**
  frameworks for reports and
       accounts, 111
  identifying epiphanic experiences,
       95–98
  identifying illuminative experiences,
       95–98
  incorporating diverse data, **110**
  interpretive analysis, 93–94
  introduction to, 90–91
  non-interview data incorporation,
       109–110
  selecting key people, 95
  significance of, 98
  terms and concepts, 102
  verbatim principle, 102
  what, who, how, where, when, why, 100
Data gathering, 43–44, 58–88
  developing insight, 87–88
  document review, 59, 78
  emergent understanding, 87
  emerging accounts, **87**
  and focus groups, 69–74
  gathering information, 59–60
  interviews, 59, 60–69
  literature review, 84–86
  look-think-act, 59
  materials and equipment, 59, 78–79
  participant observation, 74–77
  recording information, 81
  records review, 59, 78
  sources of information, 58–88
  surveys, 81–84
  triangulation, 60
Davey, N.K., 13, 49, 60, 90, 92, 120, 132
Dependability, 52
Dilthey, W., 21
Distribution of scores, and Statistical
     and numerical data, 84

Diverse case analysis, 51
Documents, and data gathering, 78
Dodds, Jacqui, 2, 143, 164
Doolittle, N., 14

Eastwood, S., 2, 143, 163
Empowerment strategies, 153–154
Engagement index of, 54–55, **55**
  apathy, 54
  excitement, 54
  interest, 54
  resistance, 54–55
Engaging people's passion, 140
Epiphanies
  analyzing of, 91–102, **94**
  and data gathering, 80–81
  deconstruction of, 98–100, **99**, 101–102
  defined, 92
  identification of, 95–98
  and illuminative experiences, 92–93
  interpretation of, 93–94
  and member checks, 97–98
  observations and representations, 100
Ethics; *See* Research ethics
Ethnographic interviews, 62
Ethnographies, 119–120
Evaluation, 148–151
  audit review, 149
  open inquiry, 148–149
  participatory, 150–151
Evocative accounts, 119
Experimental method, purpose of, 19
Experimental research, and objective
    science, 18–20
Expression, and data analysis, 96–97
Extreme case sampling, 41

Facilities, and data gathering, 80–81
Fals-Borda, O., 7
Ferketich, S., 14
Field notes
  and interviewing, 68–69
  and participant observation, 75–76
Focus groups
  and analysis, 112–113
  bringing people together, 70–71
  and data gathering, 69–74
  grand tour questions, 73
  guided tour questions, 73
  mini-tour questions, 73
  processes, **70**, 72–73
  questions for, 73–74
  task-related questions, 73–74
Focusing
  and action research, 37–39
  researchable question, 38–39

Forni, E., 136
Framing the study, 35, 39
Frus, P., 84
Fuller, R., 7

Genat, W., 92, 96, 109, 144
Goffman, E., 54
Goodenough, W., 21
Gordon, D., 14
Gould, M., 13
Grand tour questions; *See*
    Questions
Green, L., 154
Greenbaum, T., 70
Grossman, C., 178
Guba, E. G., 50, 51, 121
Gubrium, J., 61, 66
Guthrie, C., 166

Hart, E., 13
The Handbook of Research, 7
Hassell, K., 13
Hazardous waste problems, case study
    for, 166
Health promotion development
    evaluation, 156
  hazardous waste problems case
    study, 166
  implementation, 155–156
  and Internet, 188
  needs assessment, 154
  planning, 155
  prioritize needs, 155
  program development,
    154–156
Heath, Bryce, 103
Heron, John, 7, 27
Hills, M., 13
HIV, and Internet, 188
Holly, M.L., 107
Holstein, J., 61, 66
Horowitz, I., 45
Hospitals, creative prevention
    strategies, 167
Huffman, J., 157
Human interaction
  and action research, 32–35, **34**
  and Australian Aboriginal people,
    23–24
  and qualitative research,
    20–25

Illuminative experiences, 92–93; *See
    also* Epiphanies
  identifying of, 95–98
  interpretation of, 93–94

Inclusion, 56
Incontinence
  managing, 8–9
  self-care strategies in community
    nursing, 163
Index of engagement, 54–55, **55**
  apathy, 54
  excitement, 54
  interest, 54
  resistance, 54–55
Information and data sources, 35,
    43–44; *See also* Data analysis;
    Data gathering
Informed consent, and research ethics,
    46–47
Ingestible, 105, **106**
Inquiry audit, 52
Institutional reports, 40
Institutions, and ethical protocols, 46
International organizations, and
    Internet, 187
Internet
  action research guidelines and
    methodology, 185
  alcohol and drugs, 188
  and community health, 187
  community organizations, 186
  general resources, 184–185
  government-sponsored web sites,
    186–187
  health promotion, 188
  HIV, 188
  international organizations, 187
  mental health, 188
  on-line web searches, 183–184
  university programs, 189
  useful websites, 184
  women's health, 185–186
Interpretive analysis, 93–94
Interviewing
  ease of, 63–64
  ethnographic, 62
  field notes, 68–69
  guided conversations, 60–74
  initiating of, 61–62
  member checking, 69
  questioning techniques, 62–67
  recording information, 67–69
  relationships of trust, 61–62
  tape recorders, 69
  verbatim record, 68–69

Jackson, M., 21
Jamault, M., 176
Janson-Bjerklie, S., 14
Johnson, J., 19, 53

Joint accounts, 121
Joint and collective accounts, 120–122

Kastern, H., 107
Kellner, 20
Kelly, A., 2, 32
Kelly, S., 143, 163
Kemmis, S., 7
Kent, J., 13
Kincheloe, J., 54
Kitzinger, J., 70
Koch, Tina, 2, 8, 9, 143, 144, 163
Komaromy, C., 13
Kralik, Debbie, 2, 8, 9, 143, 144, 163
Kretzmann, J., 167
Krueger, R., 70
Kvale, S., 61, 66

Lather, P., 53
Lee, L., 7
Lewin, G., 7
Lewin, K., 7
Life-world, 20–22
Lincoln, Y.S., 49, 50, 51, 121
Literature
    deconstructing the literature, 85–86
    including information from, **85**
    institutional reports, 40
    perspectives, 41
    practice literature, 40
    preliminary review of, 40–41
    primary sources, 40
    process of reviewing, 85–86
    professional literature, 40
    review of, 84–87
    search, 40–41
    secondary sources, 40
    using the review, 86
Lomax, P., 7
Look-think-act research cycle, 36, 59,
        90, 139–140
    adaptation of, 143
Luckman, 20
Lupton, C., 1, 13

MacKenzie, A., 13
Malinowski, B., 66
Maltrud, K., 148, 150
MAP; See Multi-disciplinary action plan
        (MAP)
Marcus, George, 27
Mascarenhas, J., 73
Mash, B., 179
Materials, and data gathering, 80–81
Maximum variation sampling, 41
McClaren, P., 54

McCracken, G., 61, 66
McCurdy, D., 60
McElroy, A., 175
McKenzie, Dr. Ray, 2
McKnight, J., 167
Mcleod, D., 177
McNiff, J., 7
McTaggart, R., 7
McWhinney, I., 141
Medical sociology, 60
Member checks, 52
    and epiphanies, 97–98
Menon, M., 180
Mental health, and Internet, 188
Merriam-Webster online dictionary, 3
Meulenberg-Buskens, I., 179
Mienczakowski, J., 13
Milgram, S., 45
Mini-tour questions; See Questions
Mission statements, and strategic
        planning, 158–159
Moon, G., 1, 13
Morgan, D., 13, 70
Moyer, A., 176
Multi-disciplinary action plan (MAP),
        141, 142
Munn-Giddings, 13

Narrative accounts, 119–120
Naturalistic inquiry, 4, 16–17
    and human social life, 20–25
    interpretive approach, 24–25
Nicolaas, G., 13
Noffke, Susan, 7, 14
Non-experiments; See Quasi-
        experiments
Nursing practice
    changes to, 13
    process of, 141–143
    self-care strategies, 163
Nursing process, 141–143
    analysis, 141
    assessment, 141
    case management, 143
    diagnosis, 141
    evaluation, 142–143
    implementation, 142
    planning, 142

Objective of studying, 28
Objective science, 4, 16–20
    and experimental research, 18–20
Occurrences, and Statistical and
        numerical data, 83
O'Hagan, M., 176
Oleson, V., 53

Oliver, S., 1
Open inquiry evaluation; See
        Evaluation
Operational plans, and strategic
        planning, 159
Ottawa Charter on Health Promotion,
        28, 151

PAR; See Participatory Action Research
        (PAR)
Participant debriefing, 51
Participant observation, 74–77
    field notes, 75–76
    photographs, 76–77
    recording observations, 75–76
    tape recording, 76
    video recording, 77
Participant, sampling and selecting of,
        41–43
Participation, 56
Participatory Action Research (PAR),
        8, 26, 28
Participatory evaluation, 150–151
    steps for, 150–151
Participatory validity, 53
Patient-Centered Clinical Method, 141
Pattison, S., 13
Peckham, S., 1, 13
Peer debriefing, 51; See also
        Participant debriefing
Peersman, G., 1
Permissions, and research ethics,
        45–46
Persistent observation, 50–51
Petch, A., 7
Petty, R., 92
PHC; See Alma Ata Declaration on
        Primary Health Care (PHC)
Phenomenology, 24
Photographs, and participant
        observation, 76
Planning and design, 35–44; See also
        Research design
    building a preliminary picture, 35, 36
    data analysis, 35, 44
    data gathering, 35, 43–44, 58–88
    ethics, 35
    focusing, 35, 37–39, 44
    framing the study, 35, 39, 44
    information and data sources, 35,
        43–44, 58–88
    institutional reports, 40
    literature search, 40–41
    look-think-act research cycle, 36
    objective of studying, 28
    practice literature, 40

preliminary literature review, 40–41, 44
primary sources, 40
professional literature, 40
researchable question, 38–39
research ethics, 45–48
secondary sources, 40
selecting participants, 35, 41–43
validity, 35, 48–54
working principles for, 55–56
Planning, and problem solving, 144–147
Polacsek, M., 148, 150
Positivism, 16; *See also* Objective science
Poverty & Race Research Action
        Council, 186
Practice literature, 40
Practitioner researchers, 10
Pragmatic validity, 53
Prattis, J., 132
Presentations, 126–131
    audiences and purposes, 127
    audio-visuals, 129–131
    body of, 128
    conclusion, 129
    enhancing verbal, 129–131
    interactive, 131
    introduction of, 128
    planning of, 128–129
Presentations; *See also*
        Communication; Reports;
        Written reports and accounts
Prevention strategies, hospitals and the
        community, 167
Primary sources, 40
Problem solving
    action planning, 144–147
    creating pathways, 145–146
    investigating alcohol issues, 168–169
    matrix for, **169**
    planning chart, **146**
    reviewing plan, 146–147
    setting priorities, 145
    supervision of plan, 147
Professional development, 156–157
Professional literature, 40
Prolonged engagement, 50
Prompt questions; *See* Questions
Public Citizen Health Research
        Group, 186
Public involvement, 13
Punch, M., 45
Purposeful, and sampling, 41–42
Purposive sampling, 41–42

Qualitative research, 4, 16–17, 20–25;
        See also Naturalistic inquiry
    and human social life, 20–25

interpretive approach, 24–25
    and preliminary literature review, 40
Quality, and action research, 48–49
Quantitative research, 16
    and preliminary literature review, 40
Quasi-experiments, 19
Questions; *See also* Data gathering;
        Interviewing
    encouragement, 66
    example, 66
    extension, 66
    and focus groups, 73–74
    grand tour, 62–64, 73
    guided tour, 73
    mini-tour questioning processes, **65**
    mini-tour questions, 64–65, 73
    phase one, 62–64
    prolonged engagement, 67
    prompt, 66
    recording information, 67–69
    and surveys, 82
    and tape recorders, 69
    task-related, 73–74
    techniques for, 62–67
    tell me about, 62–63

Rahman, M., 7
Reason, P., 7
Records, and data gathering, 78
Referential adequacy, 51–52
Relationships, 55
    and interviewing, 61–62
Reports; *See also* Communication;
        Written reports and accounts
    construction of, 123–126
    data review, 123
    define audience and purpose, 123
    format of, 126
    framework of, 126
    identifying elements of experience, 124
    member check, 125
    participant perspectives, 123
    review and edit, 125
    significant features identification, 124
    writing of, 124–125
Representation, 115–136; *See also*
        Communication; Reports;
        Written reports and accounts
    communication, 117–118
    introduction, 116
    written reports and accounts,
        118–126
Research; *See* Action research
Research about practice, 32
Research design, 35–44; *See also*
        Planning and design

building a preliminary picture, 35, 36
data analysis, 35, 44
data gathering, 35, 43–44, 58–88
ethics, 35
focusing, 35, 37–39, 44
framing the study, 35, 39, 44
information and data sources, 35,
        43–44, 58–88
institutional reports, 40
literature search, 40–41
look-think-act research cycle, 36
objective of studying, 28
practice literature, 40
preliminary literature review, 40–41, 44
primary sources, 40
professional literature, 40
researchable question, 38–39
research ethics, 45–48
secondary sources, 40
selecting participants, 35, 41–43
validity, 35, 48–54
working principles for, 55–56
Research ethics, 45–48
    agreement to participate, 47–48
    confidentiality, care, and sensitivity, 45
    informed consent, 46–47
    institutional ethical protocols, 46
    permissions, 45–46
Research facilitators, 10
Researchable question, 38–39
Researchers, 10
Ricoeur, P., 21
Roberge, G., 176
Rogers, A., 13
Rorty, R., 132
Rose, K., 177
Ross, F., 13
Rubin, H., 61, 66
Rubin, I., 61, 66

Sampling and selecting participants,
        41–43
    extreme case, 41
    maximum variation, 41
    theory or concept, 42
    typical, 42
Sani, I., 136
Sapsford, R., 7
Scheurich, J., 49
Schmuck, R., 7
Schofield, A., 2, 143, 163
Schouten, Dirk, 77, 134
Scientific inquiry, 18–19
Scientific investigation, 19
Scientific positivism, 4, 18
Seale, C., 13

Secondary sources, 40
Selim, P., 143, 144, 178
Sensitivity, and research ethics, 45
Sewell, S., 32
Shepherd, G., 175
Sieber, J., 45
Significance, and data analysis, 98
Silver, E., 156
Smith, M., 156
Smith, S., 7
Smithbattle, L., 14
Snowballing, 43
Social Action for Health, 186
Sonnack, D., 163
Spart, S., 192
Spencer, S., 1, 7, 13
Spradley, J., 60, 62, 63, 74, 97, 100, 105
Stake, R., 51
Stakeholders, 10, 42; *See also* Sampling
        and selecting participants;
        Stakeholding groups
    identification of, 42
    index of engagement, 54–55
    joint and collective accounts, 120–122
    participatory validity, 53
    primary, 42
Stakeholding groups, 42
    index of engagement, 54–55
    selection of, 43
    and snowballing, 43
Statistical and numerical data
    central tendencies, 83
    comparisons, 83
    correlations, 84
    distribution of scores, 84
    occurrences, 83
    and surveys, 83–84
    trends or history, 83
Stein, M., 156
St Leger, A., 1
Strategic planning
    action plans, 159–160
    building of, 157–158
    framework, **160**
    mission statements, 158–159
    operational plans, 159
    vision statement, 158
Street, A., 144
Stringer, E., 7, 8, 143
Stuhlmiller, C., 14
Sumara, D., 7
Surveys, 81–84
    conducting of, 82–83
    cross-sectional design, 81
    longitudinal design, 81
    numerical data, 83–84

statistical data, 83–84
Systematic inquiry, 28
Systems of meaning, 105–107

Tape recorders
    and interviewing, 69
    and participant observation, 76
Tapitch, B., 141
Taxonomy, and categories and coding,
        105–107
Taylor, B., 7, 14, 163
Taylor, P., 1, 13
Tennant, G., 157
Theory or concept sampling, 42
Toombs, S., 22
Total Quality Management, 157
Transferability, 52
Trends or history, and Statistical and
        numerical data, 83
Triangulation, 51
Trinh, T., 132
Trustworthiness
    and action research, 49–50
    and credibility, 50–52
    conformability, 52–53
    dependability, 52
    transferability, 52
Tullo, A., 177
Typical sampling, 42

UNICEF, 8, 28, 139
Units of meaning, 105
University programs, and Internet, 189
Unsworth, J., 1, 7, 13

Validity; *See also* Trustworthiness
    and action research, 48–55
    index of engagement, 54–55, **55**
    participatory, 53
    pragmatic, 53
    and trustworthiness, 49–53
Van Willigen, 14
Ve, H., 7
Verbatim principle, 102
Verbatim record, 68–69
Video and electronic media; *See* Artistic
        and dramatic performances
Video recording
    and participant observation, 77
Vision statement, and strategic
        planning, 158

Wadsworth, Yoland, 12, 14, 27, 148
Wallerstein, N., 148, 150
Walsworth-Bell, J., 1
Wass, A., 28, 139

Waterman, H., 177
Watling, Rob, 77, 134
Web searches, 183–188; *See also*
        Internet
    general website resources, 184–185
    useful sites, 184
Western scientific knowledge, changing
        of, 13
Whitehead, J., 7
Wicks, D., 1, 13
Williams, A., 1, 13
Winter, R., 13
Wolcott, Harry, 103
Women's Health and Action Research
        Centre (WHARC), 185
Women's health, web searches, 185–186
Wong, K., 181, 182
Working developmentally, 11–12
Working principles, 55–56
    communication, 56
    inclusion, 56
    participation, 56
    relationships, 55
Workplace, enhancing of,
        143–144
World Health Organization, 8, 151,
        154, 158
    case study of, 179
Wound management, action research
        case study, 178
Written reports and accounts, 118–126;
        See also Communication;
        Reports; Written reports and
        accounts
    accumulating knowledge and
        experience, 122–123
    artistic and dramatic performances,
        132–136
    autobiographies, 119–120
    biographies, 119–120
    clinic level documentation, 122
    collective, 121
    construction of, 123–126
    ethnographies, 119–120
    evocative accounts, 119
    joint, 121
    joint and collective accounts,
        120–122
    narrative accounts, 119–120
    presentations, 126–131
    record, 122
    research, 122–123
Wros, P., 14

Yorks, L., 7
Young, S., 92